D0462710

You Don't Have To Be Dy...

You Don't Have To Be Dyslexic

Dr. Joan M. Smith

Learning Time Products, Inc.
Sacramento, California
1996

Contents

Credits

*I would like to thank the following authors and publishers for
permission to quote from their works.*

"Appalling Illiteracy." Richard T. Thieriot. Reprinted by
permission, *San Francisco Chronicle*, May 22, 1988.
Copyright *San Francisco Chronicle*.

"Can Your Workers Read?" Karen Berney. Reprinted by
permission, *Nation's Business*, October 1988. Copyright 1988,
U.S. Chamber of Commerce.

"I Had to Grow Up Fast." Ellen Hawkes. Reprinted by
permission of *Parade Magazine* and the Wallace
Literary Agency, Inc. First appeared in *Parade Magazine*,
January 8, 1989. Copyright 1989, Ellen Hawkes.

"Manley's Secret Shame." Bob Dart. Reprinted by permission, *Cox Newspapers*, Reprinted in *San Francisco Chronicle*.

Smart But Feeling Dumb. H. Levinson. New York:
Warner Books, Incorporated.

"The Perceptual Talent." R. Davis. Reading
Research Council.

Acknowledgements

For Sharing their knowledge, brilliance, creativity and commitment to make learning a joyful experience.

A. Jean Ayres
Miriam Bender
Elaine Boder
Vicki Brummel Barber
Ron Davis
Joseph Farrington
Ann Freers Murray
Marian Frostig
Michael Gardiner
Hal Hanson
Karen Hoffman
Lois Kenyon
Patricia Lindamood
Maria Merkling
H. Myklebust
Lucille Packard Foundation
Howard Runion
Cheri Smith
Jill Stowell
Mary E. Williams
Steve Watts

Frank Belgau
Eugene Black
Lucinda Bonnifield-Wolinski
Judy Basta Brislain
F. H. Duffy
Cynthia Sophia Franklin
Chilant Frenzell
Gerald Glass
Preston Gleason
R.G. Heckleman
Colleen Jones
Harold Levinson
Penny Meneni
Stephanie Morris
Samuel Orton
Sheila Ramsey
Arthur Singer
Susan Smith
Robert Valett
Rick Van Zant
Eufay Wood

Purpose

The purpose of this book is to assist parents, teachers and individuals with a dyslexic learning style to recognize their unique talents. It is important for people to understand how these talents interact to form a unique learning style. It is essential that these individuals with a dyslexic learning style utilize their learning skills to improve and increase their acquisition of information.

During the past seven years, we have learned to understand the dyslexic condition in a new way. It is no longer a mysterious condition. Individuals with a dyslexic learning style have learned to process information differently. Most of them are very talented individuals who can learn to use their talents in learning to read.

Our clients with dyslexic learning styles participate in either twice weekly tutorial sessions or intensive programs. Intensive programs were initially developed to provide therapy for clients who resided outside our community. Now they are provided for clients who want to increase their learning skills rapidly.

The information and individual case studies included in this book come from our research with these clients. The significance to their accomplishments is important for all individuals who experience the impact of dyslexia. These clients have succeeded in using their dyslexic learning style as an asset and they have learned to read.

We have identified at least three types of dyslexic learning styles. Although many of the characteristics overlap, they are readily distinguishable. A discussion of each of these dyslexic learning styles, the impact on students and the success of our clients is included in Part One, "What Does It Mean to Be Dyslexic?"

Part Two, "Remediation For Success," provides specific assessment information and training techniques for remediation of inefficient learning skills. This part of the book provides teachers and therapists with specific information about what works for each learning style. For additional information regarding the programs or services available for dyslexic learners the reader may call the Melvin-Smith Learning Center at 1-800-50-LEARN.

Introduction

The Melvin-Smith Learning Center was established in 1968 and has been helping clients with learning problems for over twenty-seven years. Over seven thousand clients of all ages, whose conditions have been caused by learning disabilities, head injuries, or dyslexia have been helped. In recent years, we have spent most of our time with dyslexia and have arrived at a number of significant conclusions.

We have concluded that the symptoms of dyslexia are actually represented by a number of learning styles created by misapplied natural talents. After refining the process for identifying these learning styles, we can identify why they prevent individuals from reading or reaching their expected level in other academic areas.

Most individuals with dyslexic learning styles cannot be taught to read through normal instructional approaches. Work must first be done to enable them to appropriately process information, so they will be ready to learn. Our work over the years, and most recently with our intensive training program, has produced successful strategies that prepare students to learn. These strategies include many of our own design, as well as some that have been developed and are proprietary with others.

Once the dyslexic learning style is addressed, the student is taught how to learn. At that point, a number of approaches may be used to teach reading as well as other academic subjects. The purpose is to give the student the ability to learn independently and not to force feed academic information that cannot be effectively retained or extended.

This book represents our effort to tell people with dyslexic learning styles that they can overcome that disadvantage and learn to read and live productive lives. It is also to give those who work with people with learning handicaps the ability to identify the dyslexic learning styles and to choose effective strategies.

Case studies are used extensively to describe these learning styles and to identify the approaches and strategies used for each style. The results we have obtained have been both astounding and gratifying. Many of our clients have wanted to share their initial frustrations and their ultimate successes, so it was difficult to choose the most appropriate ones.

Six individuals and their families were chosen to share their experiences. Representing a variety of ages and educational experiences, each one has experienced the impact of a dyslexic learning style. Using the educational programs explained in this book, each one has experienced the success of learning to read. These clients also share one other characteristic, each wanted to share their story, so that others will realize that they too can learn to read.

RICHY

Richy began his program at the age of thirty-one. After an injury prevented him from working as an electrician, he was to be retrained in a new occupation. When his workers' compensation counselor realized that Richy could not read, he requested an evaluation to determine what jobs Richy could do. Richy experienced a Visual Symbol dyslexic learning style. He did not experience words as whole units. He saw groups of letters and he knew some of the letter sounds. Since he could no longer do physical labor, it was very difficult to identify a job where he could be successful. His story about his school experiences and job history is characteristic of the nonreader.

ANNIE

Annie's story is shared by her mother. Annie is a gifted nine year old who experiences a Visual Symbol dyslexic learning style. During her first two years in school, she was very successful in hiding the fact that she could not read from her teachers. Her mother recognized her problems, but could not get anyone to understand what Annie was experiencing. Special education help was provided, once the problem was recognized. The program emphasized reading with flash cards and practicing the words over and over. Annie did not experience success and began to have many physical symptoms. She had many stomachaches, nightmares and began to wet the bed. She did not want to go to school and begged not to go to the special reading class. This mother's experiences will sound very familiar to other parents of children with dyslexic learning styles.

CARLEY

Another mother shares her story about her fourteen year old daughter. Carley has an Auditory Comprehension Confusion dyslexic learning style. Her parents guided her through third grade. At that time, they became aware that she needed a great deal of help. The school provided her with four years of special education help, after which she was dismissed from the program because she no longer qualified. She began to fail her classes without the support, but was not eligible to return. The teachers continued to complain, "she doesn't pay attention in class, she is late, she talks too much, and she doesn't have her work done." These are constant complaints about students with a dyslexic learning style.

JILL

At fifteen, Jill had experienced many years of frustration attempting to participate in her school program. She had excellent social skills and was quite embarrassed by being in special education classes. She frequently complained of being bored. This was the main clue that Jill experienced an Attention Focus Disruption dyslexic learning style. Jill describes the distress of being "off-task" and her feelings of frustration, so that others might recognize it in themselves.

SCOTT

Scott was employed as a truck driver until he injured his back. At thirty-five, he needed to select a new career and confront a problem he had hidden all his life. He could not read. When Scott found that the vocation which he had selected, computerized accounting, required reading, he no longer could hide behind his physical skills and math abilities. He needed to learn to read. Descriptions of his Attention Focus Disruption reflect the adult experience with this dyslexic learning style.

JOHN

Attention Focus Disruption can be reflected in any number of ways. John was becoming concerned that he was "crazy." His inability to control his attention disrupted his family life, his work and had caused him serious difficulty throughout school. At thirty-seven, he chose to confront his fears and do something. His success was rapid and startling.

Each of these clients has been open and candid in their revelations. For several of them, it was the first time they had admitted their fears about being "slow," "stupid" or "crazy." All of the messages they had received from teachers and other significant people in their lives were reflections of a lack of understanding about the dyslexic learning style. As they learned about their learning style, they understood that they were "intelligent," "bright" and "quite sane." They discovered their learning abilities and talents. They did not have to be dyslexic!

You Don't Have To Be Dyslexic

PART ONE

What Does It Mean To Be Dyslexic?

You Don't Have To
Be Dyslexic

Richy begins our story with a description of his experiences with a dyslexic learning style. His experiences are shared by others with this learning style.

> *It's a nightmare that haunts you and haunts you. You spend more time trying to make it right and you dream, but the dreams never come true. Most people think it's easy to read, but it's not. When you get to an age, like over twenty, it's not easy, 'cause you have lost twelve or fourteen years just flunking at school. You have common sense, since you can't have book sense.*
>
> *It's like the devil is sitting there talking to you, but you've got to get away, because if he catches you, you go into drugs and crime because it's all you've got and you've got to make it some way. You've got more people who don't have a good education who are in jail, not because they wanted to be bad. They have no choice, they wanted to survive. That goes for Blacks, Chicanos, Whites, everybody.*
>
> *Even if you have a million dollars and can't read, you are not happy. Look at the black football player who can't read or write. He's got all that money and he went to drugs and lost it all. That's why I say that. That's what not reading will do to you.*

The impact of not being able to read is significant when it prevents you from having a job. Richy continually applied for work and experienced rejection each time.

You go into a job and they see your work and they are impressed. They say, "I want to hire you. Be in my office on Monday morning to fill out the papers." So you go in on Monday and you try to fill out the papers and you can't. And you say "I can't read." And they say, "You can't work here." A person is not going to hire you on nobody's job if you can't read. He says you are a threat to the job and your coworkers. You can walk into a danger area and you can't read the sign. You might turn on or not turn on something. They can't hire you. They don't want to be liable.

I tell you all the people who can read are blessed. They can't tell you they know what you are going through because they don't. There are people that are going through this all their lives until they learn. And when they learn, they are the happiest people in the world because they have everything common sense and book sense.

It was easier for me in the first grade because you didn't have to know anything: you were going to school to learn something. So during the first and second grade it seemed kind of easy and I was real smart. It was around the time of seven or eight when we were trying to learn to read that it changed. I flunked for the first time. I flunked third grade and that kind of hurt me 'cause I came to school to be with my friends. And in third grade, I had to get another set of friends and start all over again.

Most of our clients report that they have been required to repeat at least one grade and some were retained more than one year. It is devastating to be held back and still not be performing any better than before.

I remember going back to no friends and the same teacher and I didn't want to go to school. But I went every day, that's the kind of parents I had. I had to go to school to learn. And the teachers never said anything. I was real slow then and the kids made jokes a lot. I went to school, but I started to with-draw from everybody. No friends, only family. I stayed that way until I finished school.

When I went to fourth grade, it was getting worse. I was steadily losing ground. I was trying to find ways of getting around it, but I was losing it. And the older I got, the smarter I got. I didn't buy someone teaching me something, I started teaching myself 'cause that's all I knew. I knew I couldn't learn anything in school, not that I didn't try. The teachers didn't pay attention to me. How can I say it: they pay attention only to the smart kids. You know how you got the honor roll kids, the middle kids and the dumb kids? The teachers they want to be proud and they pushed the dumb kids aside and put all their effort on the smart kids. And that left me and I stepped aside from all of them.

In the sixth grade, I flunked again. I wanted to quit school. I talked to my parents and my sisters and they wanted to help me, but I couldn't learn. I started going to these reading class-es and then they didn't know the proper way of teaching me. They wanted to hold me again after I was in sixth grade for the second time. But someone looked at my charts and said, "He ain't going to be able to read." And they sent me on to the next grade. They just kept passing me on after that. Every summer I would sit in a reading class, but they didn't know how to teach me. It still left me on my own.

The majority of individuals with dyslexic learning styles find that they have talents in other areas. Strong intellectual abilities or physical talents are common, even though they may not appear in the classroom.

I knew that one day I was going to finish school and not know anything, so I had to learn something that would hold me up. I learned to work with my hands. I learned the electri-cal business. That's when I started to wire up things, when I was thirteen. I knew that my reading and doing well in school wasn't going to get me where I needed to be, so I wanted to be tops in building class. I was number one in Cub Scouts and Boy Scouts. That's where I was trying to find my way, you know, get teachers to like me, so I could get through school, because I wasn't going to make it by being smart. I wanted to get with the teachers so they knew my problems, but even when they knew, they didn't know what to do or where to send me.

I was really on my own. I wanted to get some part time jobs, but I couldn't because my reading would act up. I saw those guys with scholarships to college and I said, "You don't have to read to do that." And I started to exercise and I got really good at football and baseball. Then in high school I had a motorbike wreck and that eliminated me from sports. That was all I really had going. I lost it, and I still couldn't read.

The experience of failure and defeat is a common occurrence to individuals with the dyslexic learning style. Even though they have constant experiences of failure, they find it difficult to accept that they really cannot be successful. It is the nagging feeling that there must be something else that causes them to seek an answer.

I never knew what my problem was. I was married and still trying to learn when my sister-in-law said she had seen a sketch in the paper about people who couldn't learn how to read and that they had dyslexia. This was about four years ago.

This was the first time I had any idea what was happening. No one ever told me. When I asked why, they would say, "You are slow!" The only explanation I ever got was I am slow. Why could I learn so many things that other people are saying is so difficult, why couldn't I learn to read? It wasn't that I didn't try, if I didn't try, I would have quit a long time ago. I never stopped.

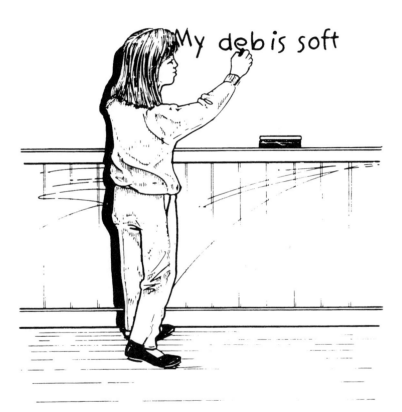

Throughout the country, Richy's experiences are repeated over and over again. Students in the schools are repeating Richy's theme every day. Men and women are attempting to get jobs and keep jobs and are repeating Richy's employment experience.

If you have a dyslexic learning style, like Richy, you are a talented individual. You do not have to be dyslexic. The way you have learned to use your mind has given you both joy and frustration. You can use your mind to learn with symbols, to read, to understand what you read, to spell, to hold the words still and to keep your attention. It is now your choice to learn to read.

Our clients share the same complaints about their frustrations in learning. The following is a list of these common complaints.

BACKWARD READING OR WRITING
Some individuals with this unique learning style have learned to read and write upside down or backwards. One young woman recalled her family physician telling her mother, *"Well, she can't read standing on her head, so somebody better teach her a different way!"* This is consistent with the classic dyslexic symptom of confusing the b and d letters. It is very difficult to read when the symbols appear to change and look different each time.

WORDS MOVE ON THE PAGE
Some individuals experience words moving or escaping them on the page. A young man described the words as *"swimming"* when he tried to look at them. Another complained that he read the same line several times before realizing that he was rereading it. Tracking from one line to another is often difficult.

CONFUSED SEQUENCE OF LETTERS
Others become so discouraged with trying to read and remem-

ber the order of the letters that they give up. They report, *"The letters look different each time I see the word. 'For' and 'of' look the same and I never know which one I am really seeing."* A common error on one of the frequently used tests for reading is the reading of "clot" for "colt." Consistent sequencing of letters is essential for reading ease.

LACK OF COMPREHENSION

Many individuals complain that they finish reading a sentence or a paragraph and have no idea what it was telling them. *"I read the whole page and then I stop and I say, 'What was that about?' and I admit: 'Damned if I know!'"*

ORGANIZATION AND TIME CONFUSION

Some find it difficult to organize materials for school and work. Some individuals experience time confusion. One mother complained about her daughter, *"She hasn't the foggiest idea that she is late. It's as though she has no sense of time passing. She can't seem to organize her books and assignments or to bring home everything she needs. She is always in trouble at school because her assignments are late. Each time she misses a deadline, she seems genuinely surprised."*

DIRECTION CONFUSION

Other individuals feel very confused at trying to understand direction and space. *"It doesn't seem to matter how hard I try, I still get confused about where to turn or which direction to go when I am trying to get to a new place. Sometimes I get lost just trying to go somewhere I have been many times."*

DIFFICULTY IN LISTENING

Many individuals have difficulty in understanding verbal instructions or listening for information. *"About the time the professor begins his lecture, my mind starts thinking about something else, and I am not aware of what is being said until he has finished."*

All of these individuals are referring to the same frustration: they have a challenge in controlling their minds. They have the motivation to be successful and correct. It does not matter how many incentives they are offered to be successful, to pay attention, to understand a paragraph or to spell a word. Their minds work in a different way, and they have little control. The way the dyslexic individual has learned to use his or her mind is unique. Each child brings a totally unique collection of talents and perceptions to the school experience. Each school experience is different and adds to the complexity by shaping the learning style for the individual.

TYPES OF DYSLEXIC LEARNING STYLES

VISUAL SYMBOL CONFUSION
The most common and earliest recognizable type of dyslexic learning style is **visual symbol confusion**. This is usually recognized at the time the child enters school and begins to learn to read. Parents and teachers both experience the frustration along with the child. They comment, *"She seems so bright and has always done well at everything. What could be causing her not to learn to read?"*

Parents initially feel that the school is not teaching correctly. Complaints from parents about the reading system are common as they attempt to explain why their "intelligent" child is not learning to read. They state:

"The school should be using a phonics program."

"The teacher needs to use a literature-based program so my daughter will be interested in learning to read."

"The teacher embarrassed my son in front of the class when he made a mistake and now he refuses to try."

"The principal said we should use flash cards at home to teach the spelling words but it isn't working."

In reality, none of these complaints explain why the child is not learning to read, nor would they make any difference in the reading development of the child. As we listen to the description about how the client with **visual symbol confusion** learns, a profile emerges.

Observations of visual symbol confusion:
1. Often confuses the b/d symbols, and sometimes 6/9, 5/2, h/y, m/n, and others.
2. Memorizes the spelling words for the Friday test, but can not recall them by the next week.
3. Likes to talk a lot, enjoys telling stories, takes charge verbally.
4. Seems to understand concepts quite easily and remembers about past events and places.
5. Interchanges words like *ran* for *run, how* for *who* or *own* for *won*.
6. Confuses words that look alike and have no associated visual imagery such as: *the, there, that, when, where, a* or *an*.
7. Confuses left and right and often has trouble copying information onto the paper.
8. Acts inquisitive and often creative.
9. Reads some long words like *birthday, elephant, television,* or *bicycle* which have different and unique patterns.
10. Memorizes stories by using picture clues, sometimes can even appear to read the story.
11. Recognizes a word in one line, but has never seen it before, in the next.

These individuals usually have specific and identifiable talents for recalling what they see when it is concrete or pictorial. This talent for visualization seems to develop at an early age.

Often described as "seeing in dimension," these individuals see an object from all sides. They seem to understand spatial concepts intuitively and perceive visual relationships in dimension. Many enjoy using this creativity in putting things together or taking them apart as they explore their environment. Others have a natural gift for drawing or building. The significant aspect of this learning style is that the individual attempts to use this "seeing in dimension" talent when he or she starts to read. When he looks at a letter, he tends to perceive it from different angles, causing him to record different images of how the letter is oriented in his mind. When he attempts to retrieve or match it, the images appear to be the same for several different labels. For instance: *If the image for "b" looks like d, b, p, and 6 and the image for "d" looks like b, d, p, and 6, which symbol do you make when you need to write a "b"?*

This type of confusion becomes more frustrating when whole words are involved. For instance: *If the word "saw" looks like was, saw, maz or zaw, how shall I spell it? What will you call "was" when you read it?*

Visual symbol confusion is often responsible for older students and adults reporting that words move as they attempt to read them. Obviously the words are not moving; however, the reader is attempting to see them dimensionally, and as the mind shifts from one view to another it appears that the words themselves are shifting.

This spatial confusion has been observed since dyslexia was first identified. The classic symptom which triggers the parental concern, *"Could she be dyslexic?"* has been the confusion of b and d symbols.

Individuals who experience this confusion when reading may have a severity of symptoms ranging from no recall of symbols at all to confusion with similar words. The same visual symbol confusion underlies both syndromes and can be addressed through similar techniques.

In Chapter Three, you will meet several individuals who

have experienced this type of learning style and are willing to share their frustrations and symptoms. Because it can be seen by the teacher or parent early in the school experience, it is the most commonly identified type of dyslexic learning style.

AUDITORY COMPREHENSION CONFUSION

While **visual symbol confusion** is very obvious because it can be plainly seen, the **auditory comprehension confusion** is the least apparent. It can be hidden as a variety of other problems, including lack of motivation, attention deficit disorder, behavior problems, even retardation. It emerges in the third to fourth grade, when listening to instructions and reading for information are required skills. Prior to third grade, students are provided with many visual tasks and frequent repetition of instructions. Up to this point, teachers anticipate that children will need help in understanding because they are young.

If formal education were to continue with the repetition of first and second grade, this learning style would be greatly ameliorated. However, abruptly in third or fourth grade the student is asked to "listen the first time" an instruction is given and admonished for asking to have it repeated. For this individual, this is only the beginning of frustration in gaining information.

Classroom assignments begin to require independent reading. The individual with **auditory comprehension confusion** discovers that he is supposed to read a chapter in a book and then answer questions about it. The only way for him to be successful is through multiple readings of the information and a piecing together of the content.

At this point, two responses are possible for individuals with this learning style. They can spend many hours on their assignments and complete them with only minimum success. Or, they can assume that it is not possible to be successful and engage in distracting or alternative behavior. These students become expert at forgetting assignments and avoiding homework, or distracting with inappropriate behavior. *"Maybe I'm too stupid to do it,"* becomes a common refrain. Even parents will confess to doubting their child's ability, even though they have evidence to the contrary. In truth, the individual is not receiving verbal messages sufficiently to respond with full information. This is evident in the frequently seen learning behaviors of this dyslexic learning style.

Observations of auditory comprehension confusion:
1. Reads words accurately but comprehension reading levels remain several years below grade level.
2. Imitates rhythms with difficulty, such as clapping out a pattern or moving to a consistent beat.
3. Engages in imagining and seems to "get lost" in daydreaming.
4. Tends to complete visual tasks very quickly, although shows no evidence of monitoring or reasoning the task through and may make many errors.
5. Frustrates easily and is hurt by others when treatment is   perceived to be unfair.
6. Tends to "track" very rapidly in reading and then misread words and lose the place.
7. Cannot synthesize or explain what was read.
8. Experiences stress in trying to explain thoughts and behaviors and often gives up, shrugs, or says *"never mind."*
9. Appears to be easily confused by verbal instructions and time schedules such as: *"You need to be home by 5:00 for dinner."*

This child has remarkable skills in putting up with a confusing world. The information he hears is inadequate and often inaccurate. As a student, this individual frequently either gives up or acts out. Since he operates without all the information, it is very easy for him to assume that what he reads in body language is the intended message. When he starts to listen, he usually fills in the blanks in the message and reacts to his own construction of what is being said.

Many students are teased about their failings as they go through school and they react in anger. They are then labeled and treated as problem students and moved through the system with little sympathy or knowledge of why the problems have occurred. It is the *hidden* nature of this unique learning style which causes them to be misunderstood.

As adults they are still confounded by the same processing problems. It is interesting that it is this group that we see most often for remediation. The same fortitude which made them survivors in the school system gave them the strength to risk getting help as adults.

A large number of adults who completed school with moderate success have this same learning style. When they experience stress, such as divorce or change in the work place, they often find that their ability to cover for their processing problems is diminished. They find it necessary to seek help and discover that it is the learning problem which is creating the stressors. Students who move from a comfortable high school environment into a large, intense or demanding university setting may also experience **auditory processing confusion** symptoms. Many adults have never identified their problem. They feel lost and confused as to why it takes them so much more energy to do what comes so easily and naturally for others. They almost always recognize this learning style and experience relief and success with interventions.

ATTENTION FOCUS DISRUPTION

The most commonly noticed and least understood of the dyslexic learning styles belongs to the individual with **attention focus disruption**. These individuals are frequently identified as being hyperactive or having attention deficit disorders (A.D.D.). The difference is that attention focus disruptions almost always are associated with efforts to work with symbols or to listen. In other words, when these students start to work on a written assignment or read information, their attention appears to wander. It also wanders when they are listening to someone give instructions or explain something.

Learning with disrupted attention focus is a challenge. The individual is not aware when he or she has ceased to attend. The child with this condition usually appears startled when called upon or when reminded she is not listening. Therefore, the wandering of attention is not a conscious choice, but rather occurs naturally as more attractive stimuli, internal or external, distract the individual.

Students with this difficulty are very frustrating to both teachers and parents. They appear to choose not to pay attention to instructions or listen for information. They often shift their focus right in front of the speaker and appear to move their eyes up, often to the left, as they engage their visualization facility. Many of them report that they start to listen to information and it makes them think of something else, and they are gone. Others describe listening as *"boring."* **Attention focus disruption** includes many readily observable traits.

Observations of attention focus disruption:

1. Enjoys creating visual images and pictures and can spend long periods attending to internal visual stimuli and dialogues.
2. Finds it very difficult to concentrate on a paper/pencil task and tends to distract within thirty seconds to two minutes, even when the task is very important.
3. Can work and stay on task reasonably well in a one-on-one activity or with computer activities.
4. Listens, thinks and carries on a conversation all at the same time, frequently making assumptions about what is being said.
5. Finds both reading comprehension and the recall of verbally presented information frustrating.

6. Likes to solve problems and figure things out. Creative talents often allow them to experience solutions without step by step (linear) thinking.
7. Does not enjoy reading and academic skills appear related to interests.
8. Tends to be impulsive and accident-prone. May break things without meaning to and is surprised at own clumsiness.
9. Likes to be the center of attention and to be in charge. Can be quite entertaining and interesting to children and adults alike.

The individual with **attention focus disruption** is frequently mis-diagnosed during the school years. Actual awareness of the true problem surfaces only during the adult years, when the individual can explain what he or she is experiencing. These individuals tend to be highly intelligent. They have strong intellectual abilities because they process many types of stimuli at once. They are frequently critical of their many skills because of their frustration in harnessing their talents for effective production.

Adults with this learning style often find success in the visual arts, construction trades, decorating, or architecture. These vocations allow them to make the most of the ability to visualize creatively and downplay the need for concentrated listening skills. There are many successful entrepreneurs with **attention focus disruption.**

Since these individuals have strong visualization skills and low verbal processing skills, they tend to experience an erratic reading pattern. They make many of the same reading errors seen in the other dyslexic learning styles. The important characteristics of their profiles are the strong intellectual ability and the capacity to process multiple areas at once. They will often complain of difficulty in concentrating and of being distracted easily.

This learning style responds very rapidly to intervention. Since these individuals are highly intelligent, once they recognize what is happening, they can quickly understand how to process and control their active minds. They enjoy the power it gives them, which enables them to adopt the new skills quickly.

PHENOMENON OF ACCEPTANCE

It is essential to recognize one other factor which complicates these profiles, the **phenomenon of acceptance**. Too often students become complacent about their inefficient and ineffective learning style. When children learn that reading or writing or studying is hard, they develop many ways of coping with their frustration or disappointment. It is as though the individual has experienced the frustration in learning and decides, *"Oh, well, that's the way it is."*

We see this time and again with children who have been through many different programs or therapies. It is likely that they had good energy and hope early in their learning, but it has long since withered and died. They have the attitude that learning is to be endured.

In our therapeutic work, we find that this phenomenon can be difficult to recognize. It does not show up during the early stages of therapy except that we find that the expected changes miss their target dates. The efforts for enduring the process require them to be cooperative and to appear to be trying. When that pattern continues after multiple hours of therapy, we begin to ask questions:

What kind of changes do you expect to see from our work together?

What would you like to do if you had the skills to do anything?

How long do you think it will take for you to improve your reading (writing, listening or whatever the goals are)?

These questions usually bring about revealing answers. The highest percentage are answered with *"I don't know"* or *"I've never thought about it."* This is a clear message that they do not believe that they can change and therefore, have accepted their learning style as a condition to be endured.

Several months ago, we encountered a young man who presented himself for testing for dyslexia. He wanted a letter written to a top university where he was enrolled to explain that he was dyslexic and needed modifications in his academic program. It was incredible to us that he had been accepted at the university and that he had been graduated from high school with his considerable learning problems. When it was suggested to him that he did not have to tolerate his present learning style and that he could change it should he choose, he became quite irritated. He stated that it had taken him years to accept his dyslexia and he was not about to change now!

This same phenomenon is frequently found in children who have been given special education placement. They learn to like their placement because the payoff is fewer demands and reduced expectations.

Many dyslexic individuals hang on to their disability simply because it is easier than to risk failing again. Since children are usually brought to the therapy setting by parents who very desperately want them to be skilled in learning, it is important to gain the child's commitment. Counseling may be helpful in opening the child to investing energy in learning.

Chapter Two

Visual Symbol Confusion

Annie and Richy experienced a visual symbol confusion dyslexic learning style. The symptoms associated with this type of reading disability are often the most severe. Both of these clients experienced a total inability to read. They could not build a reading vocabulary. Each word had to be sounded out and they did not recognize the word even if it appeared in the next line.

Annie's story is shared by her mother whose perspective on the problems she experienced will be helpful to other parents. The observations of Annie's teachers as reported by her mother illustrate how confusing an intelligent child with a dyslexic learning style can be. Annie's mother recalls:

She talked very, very early. By a year, she would talk in sentences. She could sing "Happy Birthday" or "You are My Sunshine" and any number of other songs. She had an excellent voice and was always right on tune. Now at nine, she has a gorgeous voice.

She always enjoyed music, but her favorite activity was being read to. She would bring a book and would sit for as long as you could read. She was really into watching the pictures. You know, I never realized how unusual this was until I had two other children. My two year old is just now into "let's read a story" and singing. It makes me realize how early Annie was and how perceptive she was.

She has an incredible imagination. She could engage in elaborate creative play with her dolls. She used her imagination and set up Little Ponies scenarios all around her room. Not just one set, but five sets around her room with some at school, others at the park and some at a birthday party. She's got the whole story line going all the time. She loves to tell stories.

Her other talent is in her art work. She draws with perspective and with great detail. She has done this since she was very little. She is just as creative with her art work as she is with her verbal stories.

Many individuals with dyslexic learning styles are highly intelligent and exhibit unique talents. Apparent at an early age, their intelligence allows them to mask their confusion until they reach a grade in school where reading is required and their problem becomes apparent.

This is why it was such a shock to all of us to finally accept that she was not learning to read. No one could believe it of Annie. She was so talented and wonderful about everything she did, that it seemed impossible that she would not be able to read easily too, especially since books were so important to her.

Annie is a highly intelligent nine year old with intellectual scores in the gifted range. She cannot recall sounds that are associated with symbols. As a six year old, she confused many symbols and continues at this age to mix "b" and "d" consistently. Annie exhibits a majority of the classic characteristics of the visual symbol confusion style dyslexia.

LANGUAGE SKILLS
Annie has exceptional language abilities and her vocabulary scores are superior. Her early ability to communicate, tell stories and recall lyrics are all integrated language strengths.

DIMENSIONAL TALENTS
Building elaborate sets for her toys and imagining an entire multi-scene setting is quite simple for Annie. She draws with

perspective and readily illustrates her knowledge of the dimensional world in ways that many adults would envy.

DIRECTIONALITY CONFUSION (LEFT/RIGHT)
Annie experienced great difficulty in the orientation of symbols. She consistently confused b,d and other letters. Numerals with two digits like 14 and 41 were often misread and created frustration in her math work.

COMPREHENSION STRENGTH
An enormous sensitivity to others is very apparent with Annie. She listens to them carefully and appears to intuitively understand their feelings. She does not gain comprehension from reading for herself because of her inability to read the words, but understands readily when others read for her. This is how she amassed information and vocabulary strengths.

VERBAL LANGUAGE PROCESSING
Annie understands what she hears quite easily. Her scores on digit span (ability to repeat what she has heard) are appropriate for her age. She is stronger recalling information in context than in repeating unrelated information such as a series of numbers or words. She can easily understand directions that are given to her and accumulates good information from listening.

VISUAL SYMBOL SEQUENCING
Visual symbols continued to elude Annie. She says they *"look different"* in various places on the page. She reports that letters look different based on the symbols which are next to them. For instance the d looks different in "dog" than in "rod."

It wasn't until she was nine that Annie was able to explain this confusion in symbol processing. Between the ages of five and nine, this confusion was very frightening and her behavior was predictably reactive. Her mother's account of the kindergarten through second grade years will be recognized by many parents and adults with dyslexic learning styles.

Annie was very shy when she entered kindergarten. This was a surprise to us since she had been so outgoing and enjoyed entertaining prior to this point. Her kindergarten teacher told me, "It's not that Annie doesn't know the answer. I'm convinced that she does, but the pressure is just so overwhelming for her since she is so shy. She's just not really ready to share in class."

It must have been halfway through the school year when the teachers told us that her test scores showed that she was one of the top five kids in the class. It showed that she was really ready to read and she would be in the first reading group and we could expect big things.

During the second semester, reading was taught quite actively. Then it began to unfold. The teachers were telling me how great she was, everything was great. Actually, what was happening is every four weeks the four teachers would meet and rotate their kids. Whoever Annie had at the time would say, "You know, Annie really didn't get it. Maybe we are moving a little too fast for her." And they would move her down to the next group. Another four weeks would go by and they'd say, "She's just so shy, maybe she needs a smaller group to work with." And she'd get bumped down again and finally out to the resource teacher for extra help.

Children are very aware of the hierarchy of grouping in their classroom. Highly intelligent youngsters like Annie are often stressed by their obvious failure to progress with their group. This frequently causes physical symptoms and other stress induced reactions.

It seems that no one was explaining to Annie what was happening to her. She knew that every few weeks she was ending up with a different group of kids and yet the groups still seemed to be intact except for her. Then she was removed from the room and she didn't have any reading with the other kids. At home, we began to realize that she was abnormally stressed because she was having nightmares and wetting the bed. She would get up in the middle of the night and we would find her sleepwalking and her face would be full of anguish and stress. She began having stomachaches and asking if she had to go to reading.

Parents find that they are having to teach their child at home because the child is falling behind the rest of the class. Even with the support of an interested parent and several hours work each evening, the child does not appear to be improving.

Every day after school she would bring home the papers that we were supposed to review as good parents. When she would get home, she would hand me these papers and she had no idea what the sounds were or what the words meant. She wasn't even really sure how to work the paper. She wasn't sure if you were supposed to cross out or circle the answers or what it was about. She was unaware.

I finally went back to school and said, "There is something really wrong here." The teachers said, "Well, she does fine in school."

I worked with her at home again and finally it occurred to me that when she would get home, she would not know anything because she didn't have anyone to model. She'd say to me, "Mommy, you read it first, I'll read it next." That was finally my clue. If someone would read it first, she memorized it and could remember it for long enough to perform in class.

At this point, with six weeks to go in school, I absolutely got crazy. I said, "She is not learning anything and she is memorizing." Her teachers tried to calm me by explaining that she was just "a little shy."

Teachers see students in group situations. Sometimes, they compare the child who is very intelligent and not learning to read with other children who are not learning to read. In many cases, the intelligent child does not have as many problems. When the parent cannot gain a common understanding with the child's classroom teacher, sometimes other professionals can help the parent gain a perspective and provide the teacher with new information.

I went to my pediatrician and he did a complete workup for Annie. We saw an eye specialist, a neurologist, a developmental optometrist and then I went back to the pediatrician. He said he wanted the school to test her and he would give me a letter requesting this if they refused.

That was the encouragement I really needed. I referred her for special services. The school told me that no one in the history of the school had ever qualified for special education resource help in kindergarten. It made me feel like a real dope.

The school tested Annie and held a meeting with us to review the testing. The psychologist said, "Well, because she is so intelligent, we do have a discrepancy and she does qualify for resource help."

Two positive things happened because of that meeting. First, we found out that Annie was very intelligent and that we should plan for her as a bright child. Secondly, her teacher really turned around and instead of being against me, she was really on my side. It was a wonderful feeling to find that we weren't fighting everybody.

When a student is identified for special help, it is important for the parent to understand what kind of programming will be provided. There are unique programs which are successful for the child with a dyslexic learning style. Unfortunately, the extra help may or may not provide the specialized training the child requires.

The biggest negative was that the resource teacher was unconcerned. From the beginning, I had the feeling that she felt I was a pushy mother with a problem. Even though Annie was eligible for extra help, I was very disappointed with the program. What she got was repetition, repetition, repetition. From her spelling test and the different things we had worked on, I knew that it would not make a difference. For instance, she has seen the word "was" at least five hundred times and that is pretty good repetition, and she still didn't know that word.

I thought that now that everyone understood that she learned differently, there would be something different that they would do to teach her. I think that this has been the biggest negative throughout the whole school experience.

Annie got straight A's in kindergarten. Annie got straight B's in first grade, and she still couldn't read.

Now in second grade, she is in a classroom with thirty-two children. The teacher is stressed with twenty-five boys and seven girls—and many students with behavior problems. She made Annie stay in at recess because she couldn't finish her paperwork. When I tried to suggest that I would help her with the paperwork if she would please let her go out at recess, she became furious with me. She seemed to think that I felt it was her fault that Annie couldn't get it done. At the same time, Annie was leaving the classroom for resource help and missing class work.

Many individuals with this dyslexic learning style report that they were retained at recess and other class times. They had to stay in and work instead of playing because they were unable to complete the work in the same time period or with the same success as other students. This penalty creates many problems for the child. It interferes with their socialization opportunities and makes them different from their classmates.

Since the child cannot get the work done during the school day, it is often sent home to be completed in the evening. Consequently, the child spends all day in school without recess and then several hours each evening working on tasks they cannot do. This type of situation creates physical manifestations. We have seen an increasing number of young children with migraine headaches, ulcers and other stress-induced symptoms.

> *By this time, Annie hated reading with a passion. She was having crying fits, wetting the bed, having nightmares, night walking and grinding her teeth. She would have "I don't want to go to school" hysterics every morning, especially on Friday because that's when she had her spelling test. We decided that we should have some counseling to find out how to help her to relax.*
>
> *It came out that Annie had a very definite idea about what was going on in school. From the last part of kindergarten on, she was being moved back and then was moved off the board because she was in resource. She had a very visual picture of moving down the ranks and finally out the door, but she didn't understand why.*

Annie and her mother have provided an excellent example of what a child with a dyslexic learning style experiences in the early school years. In our clinical practice where we have seen thousands of clients over the past twenty-two years, this story is repeated daily.

In listening to Annie and her mother, we can learn much about **visual symbol confusion**. First, Annie attempted to adapt to the classroom environment with every skill she had. She assumed a quiet, shy posture which covered her confusion and allowed her to stay undetected for almost a full year. Like most children, she did not know what was different although it was apparent to her that she was not learning in the same way as the other children.

Annie's mother worked in the home and was actively involved with both the school and her children. This put her in touch early with the discrepancies between her expectations for Annie and what was happening in the classroom. Even then it was difficult for the teachers to understand what she was saying. They saw a quiet, shy child and Annie performed well within their own expectations of her. She was one of many in a group of four classes which were mixed according to ability.

When Annie was finally diagnosed as "learning disabled," the school defined her problem as relating to reading and chose a remediation model based on repetition and increased time-on-task. Annie was given flash cards for both school and home. This was an unfortunate choice for a child with **visual symbol confusion**. She could not be successful with this approach because of the very nature of her learning style. Instead, it amplified her frustration and her hatred of reading.

When Annie first came to our clinic, she openly stated that she could not read. Because Annie was highly intelligent and verbally adept, we chose to involve her deeply in her own programming. We explained what she would be doing, why we expected it to be successful, and what she could expect as she progressed.

Annie cooperated in the programming, but continued to maintain the doubting reserve adopted by children who have believed the were going to be helped and then were disappointed. Annie received intensive programming in learning to read using **Easing Into Reading** and the **Auditory Discrimination in Depth** (ADD) program. At the same time, she learned to work with her strong visualization skills while forming the letter symbols and words in clay. Clay is used for clients with good dimensional skills because it gives dimension to the symbol. We also carefully integrated Slingerland tactile and kinesthetic teaching throughout.

Gradually, Annie let herself become successful in retaining the symbols. It took at least six months of twice a week sessions before we felt that she started to trust us and began to believe in herself. At the beginning of fourth grade, she had her first 100% on a spelling test with a modified list. It was the first time she had experienced total success in recalling the words. She knew them a week later, too. She is now reading in a third grade reader and recognizing the words.

Annie has lost none of her exceptional talents in art and music. She continues to develop her talents with an art instructor and frequently brings her fine work to the class-room. Annie's mother shares her feelings about Annie's early experiences in a philosophical and yet realistic comment:

> *I hope that when we get through this, and as Annie looks back on this time in her life, that she would somehow come to see it not as a downfall, but as a challenge. That it would somehow encourage her or give her the strength to know that she can achieve whatever she wants to achieve. She talks emphatically about being a pediatrician. My husband and I have talked about financing her through medical school or whatever, and I just think, I know, she could do it. I just want her to be able to feel like, whatever she decides, she can do!*

It does not matter how old the individual may be, the stress of a dyslexic learning style is part of each day. Annie was fortunate that she was just in second grade when her unique learning was identified. She could receive assistance and use her skills throughout her school years. Richy was not identified during his school years. Annie was a nine year old when we first met her, while Richy was twenty-nine.

Richy was working as an electrician on a high voltage platform when it exploded and sent him thirty feet to the ground. He experienced multiple injuries which prevented him from continuing to do physical work. We were asked to evaluate his abilities for retraining since his physical condition prevented resumption of his electrical work. His vocational counselor suggested enrolled him in a program to learn to repair jewelry. He was frustrated with his program because he was expected to read the repair instructions, but he could not read.

Richy's testing profile was very similar to Annie's. He could not recognize more than three words, and he consistently confused many letter symbols. He had tried in grade school to learn to read, but ultimately found ways to get around it. He had graduated from high school with the help of his sisters and friends. Excellent verbal and communication skills allowed Richy to charm his way through many situations successfully.

He was very talented in his understanding of the forces of physics and the dimensional world. He worked with his father in construction and repair from the time he was five years old, and eventually he made a good living as an electrician. Now without the ability to work in his field following his accident, Richy confronted his need to learn to read. He decided that he wanted to learn to read and began to devote considerable energy in this direction.

Richy's profile is typical of the **visual symbol confusion** dyslexic learning style.

LANGUAGE SKILLS
Richy was very fluent and expressive in his communication, although he did experience numerous grammatical errors, related to his self-education.

DIMENSIONAL TALENTS
This was an obvious forte for Richy, given his early understanding of construction. Electrical repair was a natural field for him. He was fortunate to have had his father as a model and mentor since a formal education in this field would have eluded him.

DIRECTIONAL CONFUSION
At twenty-nine, Richy still could not identify the direction for many of the letter symbols, nor could he distinguish between b and d, m and n and other similar combinations. Since he avoided reading and writing, he did not have the opportunity to practice or gain recognition of letter symbols.

COMPREHENSION SKILLS

Richy learned in school through listening and filling in gaps in information from his own experience. He would anticipate what someone was going to say and respond to it. Even so, his understanding of what he heard was remarkably astute. He enjoyed listening to radio and television and gained good information from both. He would obviously have good comprehension skills for reading if he could decode the words.

VERBAL RECEPTIVE SKILLS

Richy gained most of his information through listening which was a comfortable area for him. He participated easily in conversations and presented himself in an educated manner.

VISUAL SYMBOL SEQUENTIAL MEMORY

This was Richy's nemesis. He could not distinguish one symbol from a similar one and once they were embedded in words they looked different. He could not understand how they could be remembered and used to read. He could not distinguish letter names from letter sounds. When he attempted to provide a label for the symbol, he could not recall which label, sound, or letter name to use.

It was apparent that it was not a viable option for us to quickly teach Richy "jewelry" words. He would not be able to distinguish between watch/wash, solid/solder, rinse/ring or any of the names of stones or settings. At best, he could develop a pictorial dictionary with the words next to it and look up each word through a matching process.

Richy wanted to learn to read and while his workers' compensation insurance could not support teaching him to read, it would provide him with a beginning. He worked diligently at the task. He learned through a tactile/kinesthetic reading approach which utilized the **Auditory Phonics Program** and **Davis Orientation Counseling** and other programs. Clay was used for the recall of formation and discrimination of the letters. Visual logic and analysis activities were used to develop his visual discrimination skills. Richy worked intently between his weekly sessions. He had consistent stimulation and assistance by using tape recordings of his lessons.

The most dramatic change that Richy made during the first two months of his program was in his physical appearance. He radically changed his posture. He walked with his cane in a manner that made him look like a movie star. His wide smile and confidence filled the room when he entered. He was learning to read and he felt successful.

Richy was concerned when his eight year old son, living with his mother in Louisiana, was being referred for retention in second grade. He arranged to have his son spend the summer with him and attend his programming. Both of them practiced daily with the phonic drills. On the last day of the summer program, Richy filmed his son's lesson and sent it back with him for his teacher. When his son was evaluated by the school at the beginning of the fall term, the school agreed to promote him to the next grade. His teacher was so interested in the film of his lesson that she continued to work with him with the same program during the school year. Richy's son made the school Honor Roll at the end of the first semester.

It is not unusual for us to see families, like Richy's, with multiple generations of dyslexic learning styles. The pattern tends to repeat the same type of learning style. In past years, there were more work options available for the non-literate individual. We often hear family histories of grandparents who did not read, but were successful in their own businesses or farms. In today's world, the non-literate individual cannot be absorbed easily into the work force. Richy's experience brought this home to him and heightened his concern for his son.

Both Richy and Annie have visual/symbol confusion types of dyslexic learning styles. They are two very talented individuals; their skills in the arts and in construction are quite natural gifts. Their skills are related, interestingly enough, to their abilities to visualize in dimension, that same talent which made it difficult for them to learn to read. They attempted to look at the non-dimensional printed word in the same way that they looked at objects with depth; this created confusion and denied them consistent images from which to learn.

Ron Davis with the Reading Research Council in Burlingame, California describes this type of dyslexia as a tendency to disorient. His discoveries of techniques to consistently orient the way of looking at symbols has been very effective for many individuals with symbol confusion. He is responsible for educators returning to the use of clay to provide dimensional letters in remediating symbol learning disorders.

There appears to be a certain level of maturity required for learning the orientation techniques. They have been very successful with adults who disorient and bright students of fifth grade age and above. For younger students, the use of clay and development of increased attention focus have been effective in providing orientation skills. As the individuals gain skills in stabilizing the visual world, they can then begin to learn an effective reading system such as the **Easing Into Reading Program**, the **Auditory Phonics Program** or **Auditory Discrimination in Depth**.

Both Richy and Annie demonstrated the **phenomenon of adaptation**. When they discerned that reading engendered confusion and subsequent failure in their early attempts, they utilized their considerable resources to avoid print and distract their teachers and families from their failures. They developed serious fears of risking. Had Annie's mother or Richy's accident not propelled each of them respectively to find interventions, they would probably have continued a non-literate life style.

Chapter Three

Auditory Comprehension Confusion

Learning is very frustrating to individuals who have **Auditory Comprehension Confusion.** They can usually read words, but find that they cannot understand or recall what they are reading. Sometimes the confusion is not limited to reading, some clients find that they have difficulty in understanding conversations. They report that when they have to listen to instructions or an explanation of something new, they become confused or it does not seem to make sense.

This was what Carley experienced as she went through school. Her story is told by her mother and spans an eight year period. It reflects the frustration that Carley, her family and her teachers were experiencing, and it is typical of individuals with auditory comprehension confusion.

Carley was first tested in third grade for special education services. She was then provided with help through a pullout program. For an hour or more each day, she left her classroom to receive assistance with her learning problems.

In her first testing, she had a Wechsler Intelligence Scale for Children-Revised full scale score of 112. Four years later in junior high school, her full scale scores had dropped to 105. The psychological report stated that she had a *"slight decline (or regression toward the mean) in her scores since testing in 1984, but not significantly great nor was there a significant drop in any one area."*

Students in her school district must have a discrepancy of a specific number of points between their intelligence score and their academic score in order to receive extra help through special education. Because her intellectual abilities had declined, Carley no longer had the discrepancy of over twenty points. Even though she was still behind academically, she was no longer eligible for special education.

Students with **auditory comprehension confusion** frequently experience this decline in ability scores as they become older. They are not actually losing intelligence, but are not gaining new information at a consistent rate because of their listening and reading problems. Consequently, their test scores decline.

Carley had been in special education services for four years and now in eighth grade was ineligible for assistance within the schools. The meeting with the school district reported that *"There appears to be no handicap or discrepancy and Carley is not eligible for special education."*

In seventh grade, the special education teacher told Carley's mother *"She's too high for this special help class. Let's try it for a while in a regular classroom and see what happens."* Her mother was shocked that she was now ineligible for the school's support. She recalls:

> *I needed their support for Carley. You just get more support when a child's in a learning disabled class or a special education class, because they're more understanding. The teachers are more understanding and not as hard and mean on the kids...that's been my experience.*
>
> *They took her out and she fell flat on her face. Then they would not put her back. We had her tested and what was so strange was that all the tests came back stating: "This is a wonderful child one-on-one. She is very well adjusted, very happy, and has good self-esteem. I just can't understand why she's failing." And they'd say, "Well, she needs organizational skills and she needs to buckle down." And all the time I'm thinking, if you only knew how hard this child works.*

Carley has a profile typical of the individual with **auditory comprehension confusion**. With parental assistance, she was able to keep up through third grade. Then she began to have serious problems in learning. Any time she had access to one-to-one or small group instruction, she could maintain a reasonable learning level. She relied on someone to "interpret" what she had to know. She did not have the skills to listen and recall information which was not edited and demonstrated for her.

One of the most unique aspects of the **auditory comprehension confusion** is that this learning style interferes with the understanding of instructions delivered to a group. The difference between one-to-one and group delivery is critical in understanding the limitations of this learning style. When we speak with someone one-to-one, we adjust what we are saying by reading their body language. If they appear to indicate that they understand what we are saying, we go on. If they look confused or do not seem to be registering what we are saying, we repeat or restate it. This is part of the natural flow of listening/speaking.

Group instruction is quite different when the group exceeds several individuals. We can no longer read the understanding level of each person without interrupting ourselves. Therefore, we tend to speak to the group and modify our presentation based on their perceived reception.

This was the major difference in the instruction at school or at home which allowed Carley to understand or to fail. She could work at home with the one-on-one instruction or in the special class with assistance by the teacher or aide. When this support was removed, she could not comprehend the information or directions. This created stress which prevented her from using her attention skills to maximum level. Given her learning profile, failing grades should have been anticipated.

In her profile, Carley shows the strengths and weaknesses typical of the auditory comprehension confusion learning style.

LISTENING SKILLS
Carley has consistently had problems with her listening skills. She can not recall directions and frequently has to ask other students to repeat the directions. She does not remember more than a few instructions at a time.

RHYTHM SKILLS
Although Carley takes jazz dance, her mother describes her performance as a *"burst of energy."* She is not skilled in repetition of a rhythm or in maintaining rhythmic patterns.

NON-VISUAL WORDS CONFUSION
Words which convey direction such as: what, where, that, then, for and of are readily confused. She does not appear to read them and becomes quite confused in trying to deal with written directions. She can pronounce the words correctly most of the time, but the meaning eludes her.

DISSYNCHRONY IN COORDINATING VISUALIZATION AND LANGUAGE PROCESSING
Carley's eyes track rapidly across the print at a pace far different than her interpretation of language can maintain. She is often looking on the next line while her inner voice is still interpreting information on the previous line.

TRACKING CONFUSION
Carley often reaches the end of one line and again tracks the same line or she may skip the next line. She experiences such confusion in understanding what she is reading that she has difficulty in moving across the page, maintaining a continuum, and retaining information.

RAPID VISUAL PROCESSING
Carley takes in visual information quite rapidly. She assesses situations with ease and reads people and situations skillfully.

VISUALIZATION SKILLS
Creative visualizations are Carley's forte. She can develop pictures with depth, color and composition. She excels in her art classes.

LANGUAGE SKILLS
Carley's vocabulary skills are below her age level expectation. She expresses herself easily, but has not continued to develop her content or receptive skills commensurate with her other abilities.

TIME AND ORGANIZATIONAL CONCEPTS
Carley has little concept of the passing of time. She is often late to class, frequently has the wrong materials, and has no idea when assignments are due. She frequently receives detention notices because of tardiness and appears to have resigned herself to endure this inconvenience.

Reading, preparation of assignments and organization are her major complaints. She expresses a desire to please her teachers and family, but finds it difficult to *"do everything at once!"*

Carley's **auditory comprehension confusion** profile emerged in the third grade. It is readily recognizable as a serious processing problem. The symptoms of this learning style become apparent in her mother's recollection of Carley's early school history:

> *It started to get hard in third grade when we realized she was getting behind in school. If I had known more, I would have seen it coming even in first grade. She was having an hour of homework each night. It seemed to me it was like pulling teeth to get it done. She would be cooperative, but it seemed so hard to both of us.*
>
> *I might have noticed it earlier because when she came home from school she was dog tired. In kindergarten and*

preschool, she would come home full of energy and she just wanted to play. She couldn't wait to get outside and play with the animals she loves. In first grade, she would come home and be very irritable and sometimes she'd just go in and take a nap.

Stress often becomes apparent in first or second grade. As the student finds that they have to use extra effort to listen and understand instructions, they become exhausted.

One day, while she was in third grade, I was talking to a friend and telling her about Carley and what she was doing. She asked if I had ever thought of having her tested for dyslexia. All I knew about dyslexia was the reversal of letters, which she didn't do. But the inability to read part caught my attention.

About this same time, an incident occurred which made me go into action. In third grade they had spelling tests each week. One day the teacher was giving the instructions for setting up their papers. The teacher gave the five instructions: put your name on the top right, put the date below your name, write "Spelling" in the middle of the first line, remember your margins, and then number from one to twenty. Apparently Carley missed an instruction, so she turned to the girl next to her and said "What was the third thing? I know I'm supposed to write my name and do the numbers." And the teacher said, "Carley, leave this classroom, you are cheating."

The principal called me to school and said that Carley had been cheating in class. I was very emotional and I said "We will make her own up to anything that she does, but I don't believe that she was cheating." I know that probably every parent says this, but I knew that Carley had trouble with directions. She probably just was trying to find out the directions.

Incidents which appear unrelated to the dyslexic learning style often cause parents and clients to seek help. Carley's mother understood the relationship between her behavior and her learning. The school's accusation of cheating provided the impetus to seek help.

The integration of rhythm in learning is frequently a challenge for the individual with auditory comprehension confusion. Rhythm is experienced in many areas of learning beyond moving to a rhythm. Our language has a distinct rhythm. Individuals who miss the natural flow of rhythm in language cannot benefit from it as an aide in comprehension.

She never seemed to have much rhythm. She liked to sing and she knew the words and seemed to be on key, but did not have any rhythm. My recall of her was that in riding a bike or skating, she was just blustering through. Now she takes dancing, and she is very elegant in her movement. She can do the steps, but has a hard time remembering the sequence.

Once the tutor tested her, she found that she was right brained and should have been left handed. I took out a bunch of books from the library and read all about the Orton Dyslexia Society. The teachers I was talking to at school had never heard about these books. I offered to loan the books to them so they would understand what it was all about. They told me, "Dyslexia is just a catchall." They weren't even interested.

Obtaining recognition and understanding of this unique learning style is essential for gaining cooperation from the school. When teachers and school psychologists are unaware of the differences in learning strengths and needs experienced by individuals with auditory comprehension confusion, they often miss recommendations for appropriate programming.

The school district tested her and we went to a meeting to learn about the results. I sat through humiliation during that meeting. I explained about the testing done by her tutor, that she was ambidextrous, that she had dyslexia, poor memory retention, and that she couldn't sequence at all.

Then the special education teacher, who had been staring at me, looked at everybody in the room and put her head down and started laughing. "Ma'am," she said to me in a very condescending way, "I'm sorry. Who is this woman who tested her? I am sure that my tests are far more sophisticated than anything this woman could possibly do. There is no such thing as dyslexia and I don't know who ever told you that."

Afterwards, the principal came up and said "Take it with a grain of salt. She probably won't be here very long." And she wasn't. But she was Carley's resource teacher in the beginning. Then a new teacher came in whom Carley loved and who cared about her. He worked with her very nicely, but never used the materials or ideas that the tutor was suggesting. So we worked with them at home. We had Carley visualize the spelling words and write them in air. She used her large motor skills and small motor skills and Carley remembered the words, just like the tutor said she would.

Even though she liked the resource teacher, it was hard on her because she missed what went on in her classroom and that put her behind. She was also beginning to ask, "Am I stupid?" That's the first time when she was put in special education that she thought it because people would say things to her. Her friends were very protective of her and tried to help her.

Frequent doubts about one's intelligence confront the individual with a dyslexic learning style. Since they have good intellectual abilities, they can analyze and compare their performance with other students and observe their inefficiencies. Fortunately, many individuals with a dyslexic learning style appear to have special talents in creativity and art. This was especially true for Carley and it provided her with an area in which she could gain esteem.

Carley was experiencing success with her art. She was very artistic. She won a prize in fourth grade for a landscape. She had depth in it, just like she had studied drafting. It was three dimensional and the colors were beautiful. She used contrasting colors and complementary colors. It was so different from the other students work.

Even though a student might be identified as having a learning disability, it does not mean that the teachers and school staff will understand the impact on the individual's learning. The comments from teachers remain with students into their adult years. Since they are regarded as significant persons, the student internalizes teacher's opinions and take them as measures of their self-worth.

In fifth grade, she had a teacher who didn't believe in dyslexia. Every time she asked a question, she was told she didn't pay attention. In sixth grade, we brought in the testing reports and explained about her listening problems and gave examples. We thought we had explained it very well. And the very first week of school we were called and the teacher said "She doesn't pay attention." And I thought "Oh, here we go again." The teacher had us come in for an interview with Carley present. We walked in and she started yelling, "Carley doesn't do this and Carley doesn't do that and she didn't do this and she didn't do her homework." And here is Carley sitting there. I was absolutely dying.

Afterward, I went up to her and said. "Why did you do that? Do you think that it was good for her? She is dyslexic. Everything you said is typical of her problem. I thought you understood that."

When the teacher typed up her grade reports she said "Carley stares out the window a lot. I think she needs psychological counseling." My husband read the grade report and said, "I can't believe we have gone in and spent hours trying to explain, giving her reported materials and it is as though nothing has sunk in."

In seventh grade, Carley began to realize that she had many friends in school. She seemed happy with that. I think for her it was a turning point because she realized, "Okay, school's not so great, but I have friends and I talk to people and they like me, and so I like going."

Many people identify the challenges Carley was experiencing as "immaturity." The implication is that she will grow out of it. This does not happen. The individual continues to perform in an inefficient manner, as the demands become greater their problems become accentuated.

Carley is in eighth grade this year and she is having difficulty. She is late all the time to her classes. The first day of school she called me and said "I lost my list. I don't remember which class to go to first."

And that takes us back to when they tested her and said there is nothing wrong. They tell me her memory is fine but she can't remember which class to go to or where her list is. She's easily distracted by things and they test her for that and they say, "She isn't distracted." And they are telling me they can test all this, and there is nothing wrong with her. I don't really have a lot of knowledge about their tests, but it seems to me that they're not testing her in the right way.

The teacher called today and said "Carley is not paying attention in class, she talks too much in class, she is late, and she doesn't have her homework done." Sounds familiar doesn't it?

Auditory comprehension confusion is all but hidden from view. It is a distinct learning style usually complemented by strengths in visualization abilities. When the individual attempts to learn, he or she must take the "heard" information and process it in the mind's visual center. This can be observed when the individual looks away and up; descriptions of the student gazing out the window, which are interpreted as negative learning behavior, can actually reflect the attempt to register and explore information.

The challenge lies in the fact that when these individuals use the visual center to process, they often add creative information or become distracted by the creative aspect of their processing. A majority of those with **auditory comprehension confusion**, children and adults alike, find they experience difficulties with their attention focus as well. The difference between the **auditory comprehension confusion** and **attention focus disruption** dyslexic learning styles is that even when they have learned to focus their attention, the **auditory comprehension confusion** subjects continue to have language comprehension difficulties.

This particular dyslexic learning style is especially distressing for adults. The difficulties which Carley was experiencing in school are identical to those which can occur in the work place. The areas of stress occur in identified areas.

TIME MANAGEMENT

Missing deadlines and being late are consistent patterns for the adult with this dyslexic learning style. Their repertoire of skills does not include an intuitive sense of planning or organizing for deadlines. They are also often unaware of the passage of time.

LISTENING

Maintaining listening focus or concentration is extremely taxing. Since he or she has good intelligence, there is a tendency to jump ahead of the listener and to assume what will be said next. The ability to maintain an active listening/recording/listening/recording/listening interaction is extremely short. Actual timing of concentration spans among numerous clients shows a range of ten seconds to one minute. Also, since the individual is processing in chunks of information smaller than what the speaker is presenting, information is missed.

Most speakers use a pattern of seven to eight words before they take a breath. It is the speak/breathe pattern which allows the listener to use the listen/record pattern. When these patterns are in synchrony, the speaker speaks as the listener listens, and while the speaker takes a breath the listener records the information. For example if we use numerals to represent the words in a sentence, it will look like this:

1 2 3 4 5 6 7 Breathe 8 9 10 11 12 13 14

The listener pattern for an individual with four to five digit processing would look like this:

1 2 3 4 5   Breathe 8 9 10 11   14

Key pieces of information may have been contained in the words which were missed. The listener was recording information while the speaker is still talking. He is unaware that information is missed until it ceases to make sense. At that time the listener fills in the missing parts so that it can make sense because he cannot tolerate the feeling of confusion. This is called the threshold of confusion. If he knows about the subject he may guess correctly but he may also be incorrect. Once the information is added, the listener believes that it was actually what he heard.

CREATIVE VISUALIZATION
This is usually a strength for this individual. It is frequently developed to a high degree among artists, carpenters, architects or others in which it has been recognized and allowed to develop.

READING COMPREHENSION
A genuine dissynchrony exists between the visual processing and the language processing of information. For appropriate

understanding to take place, coordination must occur between the visual center and the language center of the mind. The individual tends to process visual information quickly, rapidly scanning the page. The language center works in a slower, more methodical, time-governed manner and does not process rapid visual input.

The mis-processing of information may be explained using the following example:

The cat ran across the covered bridge and into the tree near by. As the bird flew out of the tree, the cat lunged and missed.

The words are first recorded by the visual center of brain; then the information is transmitted to the language center. The individual may be seeing the word "tree" while the language center is just receiving the word "covered."

If the individual stops tracking and goes back to decode "covered," and attempts to continue from where he paused, he may return to the second "tree." The content is rapidly distorted: *"The cat ran across the covered bridge and into the tree, the cat lunged and missed."* If the comprehension question for this selection was, *"How did the bird evade the cat?"* the dyslexic individual might well ask, *"What bird?"*

The result of this processing style is missed and inaccurate information. This read and reread style is very frustrating and usually creates a genuine and understandable dislike of reading.

WRITING/REPORT DEVELOPMENT

Written work requires supportive language skills. The interaction between the inner voice (which appears to originate content) and the imaging of the words for recording is essential. As with the dissynchrony experienced in reading, there is great difficulty for the individual in connecting the words on the paper with the inner voice. The actual written work is often missing many words, and punctuation marks are often

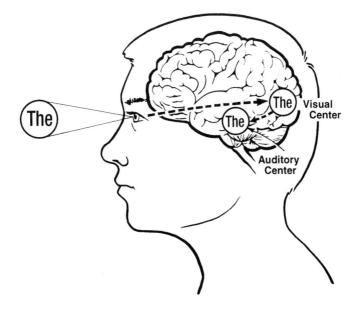

omitted. Adults with this learning style must spend considerable effort and energy to prepare a small report.

CONFUSION WITH INSTRUCTIONS
Many individuals with this learning style tend to operate their own businesses possibly because they have difficulty receiving comprehensive instructions from others. When they cannot control their own situations, they become distressed with those in charge of giving directions and change job positions frequently.

Compared to the **visual symbol confusion** learning style, **auditory comprehension confusion** is much more difficult to recognize in the school age child. Hidden from obvious view, it is often identified as a behavioral or personality problem rather than a distinct learning style. This hindrance to early identification and remediation complicates the situation. It is essential that the individual receive assistance in language processing, listening development and verbal reasoning skills. As these skills emerge, the learning style becomes a positive one and reading comprehension can begin to develop. As long as language processing is inadequate, working with reading development will be only minimally effective and the individual will continue to be dependent on an interpreter to gain information.

Chapter Four

Attention Focus Disruption

Attention focus disruption is usually found in individuals who are highly intelligent or creative. This learning style is typically confused with attention deficit disorder or hyperactivity. However, **attention focus disruption** responds to training or diet controls and does not require treatment with medication. The individuals with a dyslexic learning style who display a significant component of attention focus difficulties may be differentiated from the hyperactive/attention deficit group in several ways. First, their **attention focus disruption** tends to appear when they are working with symbol information as in reading, writing or calculating. They lose their attention focus when they work with symbols or have to listen to things which are uninteresting. Conversely, they tend to have long attention spans for tasks which are creative or interactive such as computer games. In these activities, they tend to exhibit enthusiasm, energy, and excitement. The important fact to recognize is that they *actually are attending to something else*. They are able to focus their attention even if it is not on the assignment or speaker.

One teacher referred a ten year old boy for evaluation with the statement, *"He has no attention span."* The boy was evaluated and it was readily apparent that he did experience problems in controlling his attention focus, but that he actually had strong abilities to maintain attention when and where he wanted.

In exploring the teacher's complaints with the boy, we quickly learned what was happening. The boy went to math class in a room which also doubled as an art room. She passed papers out every day and the students were supposed to begin working on them right away. He sat next to a bulletin board which displayed the art from the other class. The display changed every week, as the teacher enjoyed featuring student work. We asked the boy if he *daydreamed* in class, and he assured us that he did not. Finally, we suggested, *"You know sometimes when I am working on something and I want to take a little break, I start thinking about something else. Sometimes I even see pictures in my mind."* This caught his attention immediately and he agreed that he did that, too. *"You know in my math class,"* he said, *"the teacher has the art papers by my desk and I like to hold art contests with them. I study each of the pictures, and then I decide who has the best colors and all, and I award prizes to them. You should see their faces when they come up to the front of the stage to get their awards."*

In integrating this with the teacher's observations, everything made total sense. He was not really aware of when he "left" the math class. He apparently sat with his pencil poised over one of the first problems, looking off into space. In his reality, he was in charge of a marvelous scenario in which he was a very important art critic! He had a long attention span; he just was not focusing on the same content that the teacher had in mind.

There are at least seven characteristics which assist us in identifying attention focus difficulties:

STRONG INTELLIGENCE

This learning style requires good to superior intellectual abilities. Even if not measured on a formal intelligence test, strengths in various areas are apparent.

LACK OF EYE CONTACT

While the individual begins to listen or work with appropriate eye contact, it is usually diverted within the first minute. If the individual tends to engage visualization skills, the eyes will usually look up. If the inner voice is speaking, eyes are parallel with the ears. Eyes are usually down for emotions.

HIGH LEVEL OF CREATIVITY
Creativity may be evident in either or both the visual or auditory channel. Children are often reported to be skilled in elaborate dialogues or imaginary play. Others utilize their visualization abilities and enjoy playing with images or imagining being somewhere else.

READING INEFFICIENCIES
Unless there is a simultaneous complication with other types of learning styles, they can read anything, but cannot understand it very well. They have to reread constantly. They report that they are easily distracted as they read and often start thinking about something else.

LACK OF ATTENTION CONTROL
In understanding this learning style, one of the most significant factors is that the lack of attention control is involuntary. Individuals do not usually make a conscious decision to stop paying attention. They report that they start to use their visualization system and find that it or their inner voice just becomes a more interesting stimulus. In order of stimulus power, the printed word ranks below the verbal word.

LOSS OF TIME AWARENESS
When the attention is focused inward, the tracking of time appears to be lost. Time may appear to pass very rapidly or very slowly.

ABILITY TO PROCESS IN MULTIPLE CHANNELS
These individuals have the unique ability to process multiple trains of thought simultaneously. They describe being able to carry on a conversation with someone, be aware of who is

walking down the hall and what they are discussing, know who just answered a telephone and plan in their heads how they will finish their next assignment all at once. Adults will often report maintaining up to six active channels concurrently.

The combination of a loss of control of one's attention focus and a loss of time awareness are the most noticeable attributes of this learning style. Teachers notice the student who appears suspended in time, staring out the window or into space. We can begin to understand what goes on from the learners' perspective when we listen to them describe their experiences. One fifteen-year-old girl who has severe challenges with her attention focus and has been enrolled in special education for six years recounts:

> *You are standing there listening to your mom talking and all of a sudden she is saying, "Jill, you are not listening to me!" and sure enough I'm not. Actually, I never know I have stopped listening until someone yells at me that I'm not listening.*

Jill was not aware of refocusing her attention until something external interrupted her internal thoughts or images. She frequently described how hard it was to listen. She told her teachers, tutors and parents that things were *"boring,"* which engendered negative reactions. What she really meant was, *"This isn't making any sense to me."* One of our first goals with her was to have her verbalize what she was experiencing when she termed things *"boring."* Ultimately, she began to understand that she was not effectively processing information relating to a situation and therefore, it was uninteresting to her.

Jill was unaware of her length of attention. When she started to become aware of how long she could sustain listening before she diverted her attention, she decided it must be *"minus thirty seconds."* In fact, her attention tended to shift within thirty seconds to one minute.

Both Jill and her family began to understand that getting the instructions in class or hearing directions at home were very difficult for her. Once they understood this as being part of her unique learning style, it became much easier at home for the whole family to interact. Jill's awareness was very important because it assisted in developing her motivation to change.

Jill learned to control her attention disruption with the attention focus techniques described in Part 2, Chapter 8, "Preparing the Brain for Learning," *Attention Focus* (p.124).

Adults experience the same characteristics in learning. Our attention focus case history is of Scott, a thirty-five year old man. He had been a truck driver until a back injury forced him to select a new career. He had a great deal of difficulty accepting that he could not resume his previous job. One of the main reasons was that he knew he had a hidden problem; he could not read.

> *I knew I had some sort of reading problem, or whatever you want to call it; but being me, trying to make the best of a bad situation, I was able to do the best on my job. I felt good about the job.*
>
> *And then being hurt, the injury wasn't anything, really. The hardest part was when I found out they were going to retrain me. That's when the old fear came up, where I can't do this because I can't understand this and I can't read.*
>
> *So that's where you start getting into a lot of problems. It starts off with an attitude thing, where I don't want to be retrained to do this. I want to find something that, this will sound funny, but where there wouldn't be much book work.*

The need to find employment which does not necessitate reading is the greatest challenge experienced by adults with dyslexic learning styles. Most individuals have selected occupations in which they use their physical abilities. This alternative works more effectively for men than for women.

When performing physical labor is no longer an option, they are confronted with the limitations of their reading. Learning a new job usually requires training or schooling.

The scariest thing for me was going back to school because I remembered when I used to go to school. I remember I used to pay my sisters to do my homework for me, you know different types of homework. I used to be really good at math, so I could do all the math I needed to do, but when it came to science, geography and reading things and understanding things, I would always have a problem. Yeah, I was really afraid to jump in and do something.

Then I basically got thrown into what they selected for me: a computerized accountant. I just knew right off the bat there would be a lot of math and I could get away with that, right?

Then I got the course outline and saw all of the classes: reading, English and more. I knew I was heading for trouble. I was really bummed out. Finally, I got to the point where I knew that I couldn't let my attitude get in my way.

Many adults attempt to develop their own reading ability by using children's materials. Many purchase phonic records or other programs they hear advertised on the radio or television. The image of this mature man working with beginning children's readers and trying to teach himself to read was heartbreaking. Still he was not successful, and he was desperate to find a solution.

I knew that I had that reading problem all along, and I really wanted to have done things. I used to try to learn to read with the little kids' books. I think I still got them somewhere. My mother-in-law, who used to be a kindergarten teacher, gave me a bunch of stuff. I would read all that stuff. I really wanted to get rid of this problem. I wanted to read better and do all of this stuff and be good at it.

So I just decided that, well, I could go in and mope or I could take this opportunity and further my reading and be a lot better. And if by some miracle I could go back to driving trucks, I'd be able to read a little better, also. So I thought, "It's time to change my attitude."

Confronting reading problems takes fortitude. Most adults have hidden their problems for so long that to seek help is frightening. There is always the fear of failing. After many years of being unsuccessful in learning to read, there is a nagging fear that, *"Maybe I really can't learn because something is wrong with me."* This was a serious fear for Scott.

When I first started coming here, I felt really stupid. I had this thing about me that I felt stupid anyway because I couldn't do anything anyway. I had to get out of that and keep an open mind. Eventually I started getting better. I noticed the difference in reading. I was able to understand things for the first time. I could read things without having to read it over and over and over.

Before, I would read something, I would read a sentence. I would read one sentence, and then another, and after I read the second sentence, I wouldn't even know what the first sentence was all about. I had to go back and read it over again and try to tie the two of them together.

I finally decided, if I have to do all of that, why bother. After a while, I got to where I didn't even want to read a book or something with instructions because I wouldn't understand them anyway. I would do better just looking at the pictures than by trying to read it.

One of the important aspects of Scott's program was assisting him to maintain his attention focus. We discovered that he actually had many reading skills. Skills which he had hidden away over the years because he could not stay focused long enough to use them. He was attempting to work with a computer in a classroom with other students and he knew everything that went on in the class except what was on his screen.

I could read something and any little thing would distract me. I could go on reading and a little noise would go by and I was sitting wondering what it was. Then I would have to go back and start over in reading. When I was reading, I would understand one sentence and then read a couple more and understand another one, so it was very fragmented. When I got through with it, I didn't get anything out of it. I could read any of the words. I could read five words and tell you what each word meant, but put them together and I couldn't do it.

Keeping on track was my biggest problem. Maybe they were describing in a book where to fish. They say where the best places are and what the fish looked like and other things. What would happen is I would get to the part where they were describing and all of a sudden whatever I was reading just turned into words. My eyes may be seeing the words, but my mind is seeing what it looks like to fish. I'm starting to see boats going by me, or me fishing. I can remember everything I was reading right up to that point where they started to describe it.

Scott provides a good example of attention focus disruption This type of disruption happens multiple times in a single paragraph. It causes the individual to confuse what he is reading with what he is imagining.

For instance, if I was reading a book and an airplane goes by, all of a sudden I see myself flying an airplane. I know that you have said that it takes talent to do that, but it sure mixed up my reading. Anyway, now I can control it, and that makes it even better.

Scott responded very effectively to Orientation Counseling. It is an excellent procedure for working with adults who tend to disorient and distract themselves while they are working. This programming is described in *The Gift of Dyslexia* by Ronald D. Davis which is referenced in the Appendix.

> *Ever since we did the orientation thing, I can recognize when I am doing it and I can think about getting back on focus and I can go right back to my reading. Now, I finish reading and then go back and visualize all I want to. The most important part is, I can control it.*
>
> *You know, I am doing all right with that "staying on point." The technique is fascinating. I said to myself when she did it, "She's going to do this and next week I'll forget all about it. It's no big deal." But you know, it didn't happen. It just stayed there. And I could keep using it. It definitely helped.*

When adults begin to experience the ability to control their minds, many aspects of their lives change. They feel better about themselves and this increase in self-esteem shows.

> *Before, it was like I was always down on myself. I've been like that all my life. I have always been harder on myself than anybody else has. I felt like I was ugly, I felt stupid.*
>
> *But now, I find I'm full of joy and more happy about things. Even though things happen, I can deal with myself more now. I know that if you really want something, you can get it. I feel I can do it. I'm in charge of me!*

Scott has now been asked to teach the class in computerized accounting that he had been taking. He had become very skilled in his course work and enjoyed being the teacher.

Gaining control of the attention focus is the key to effective learning. As long as the attention disorients, there is no opportunity to process external information efficiently. These individuals cannot stay attentive long enough to learn new information.

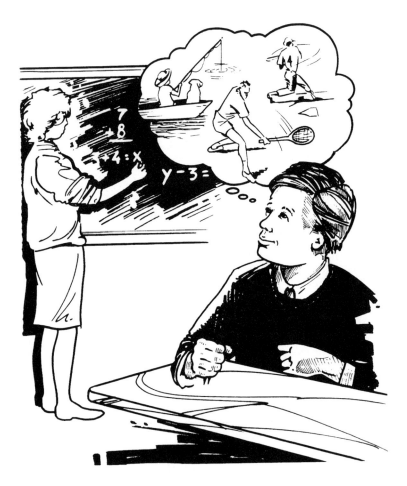

An eight year old boy was enrolled in our intensive program (three hours daily of individual therapy for four weeks) for attention focus training. Our initial impression of him was that he was very scattered. He exhibited many of the signs of classic hyperactivity. He experienced a disrupted home life and had been in home schooling for the previous six months after a very unpleasant and possibly abusive school experience. We had to establish a behavior modification program with frequent rewards to keep him on task long enough to test him. Even then, his attention span was less than one minute and during the assessment it deteriorated further.

It was clear that he really wanted to learn to read. He talked about it during his testing. He talked about the books he had and how he was going to learn to read after he came to the clinic. He had the mistaken impression that the testing was going to teach him to read.

At his age, the most effective attention training program involves using the balance beam or balance board as described in Part 2, Chapter 8, "Preparing the Brain for Learning," *Perceptual Motor Attention Training* (p. 129). During his first sessions, he could stand or move on the balance beam for less than ten seconds before he had to step off. We found that when he worked on it with his shoes off he appeared to have greater sensitivity to the surface and maintained his balance more effectively.

By the third day of his intensive program, his attention focus seemed unchanged. He had, however, started holding new information. He also took keen delight in sharing with each tutor what he had learned from the previous tutor.

As he was working on the balance beam the fourth day, his clinician observed that he seemed to lose balance and fall over for no apparent reason. We had seen similar behaviors in others and were concerned that we might be seeing some part of a petit mal seizure pattern. We decided that the clinic staff member who was with him the next time he fell over should

ask him what he was experiencing. The opportunity presented itself for one of his clinicians that same day.

His clinician asked, "What are you doing?"
He responded, "Oh, I left my body and I fell over."
She said, "Can you get back in it?"
"Sure, that's easy," he replied.
"All right, then I want you to get in your body and look out
through your eyes and keep your balance," his clinician
responded.

He did exactly that. From then on, whenever we wanted
him to return to his attention focus we asked him, *"Are you in*
your body?" or instructed him to *"Look out at this through your*
eyes." He proceeded to do a two minute, thirty-five second
attention focus, moving easily on the balance beam. He was so
excited he had to show everyone he could find, over and over
again. We all cheered his success.

This was the turning point. He began to move in his reading with startling speed. It seemed that he already knew many
words and what he gained was the ability to retrieve them. He
was taught a reading system with a phonic base and has continued to learn at an appropriate pace.

It may sound very strange to talk about "getting back in
your body." This is not a reference to a psychic experience or
phenomenon. When we visualize information, we can image it
as being internal (inside our head) or external. He tended to
image things visually out of his body and to the upper right.
When we engage in this behavior, it tends to disrupt our balance point. If while he was on the balance beam, he started to
change his attention focus to a creative visualization, it caused
him to lose balance. Achieving the control over an active visualization system is often quite difficult. In the following case
history, we can see the frustration and chaos that an individual
with the inability to control attention focus can experience.

John works at a job in which he makes deliveries to homes and businesses. He is paid by the number of deliveries he makes in a period of time. He has an excellent knowledge of the city and the addresses. He has excellent visualization skills. He can visualize his route for the day and prioritize his deliveries to maximize his time.

John came to us with a complaint about his reading, but he was even more concerned about the feeling that he was losing control of his mind. He had been under a great deal of stress and seemed to be dealing with what he described as the *"wild thoughts of my third eye."*

When John had an argument at home in the morning, it would stay with him throughout the whole day. While he was driving his route he would see a replay of the morning's incident. He continued his argument with active visualizations. This behavior had a direct impact on his work. He found that he went right past his stops, missed his turns, and had to double back, slowing his deliveries and costing him money. It also was frightening to him because he was not certain that he could control these *"wild thoughts."* John shared his experiences for us:

I was experiencing dissatisfaction in my reading. I had difficulty in understanding certain things that were presented to me. The difficulty was that my concentration wouldn't be into the reading. I couldn't control my third eye. Learning to be 'on point' has helped me a lot as far as helping to control these wild thoughts of this third eye.

It was really hard to concentrate on what was before me. I would feel my eyes blur and feel a real apprehension from past experiences in reading, especially if it entailed reading out loud with other people.

It would seem real awkward because I was thinking I would make a mistake and in most cases I would, because I perceived myself making it. I could recognize what the mistake was in advance. I just knew that I would do it. Then I got a different kind of meaning out of the sentence. I would rearrange the sentence to a certain extent. I'd drop out a word or not even know what a word was. I had a lot of difficulty with trying to phonetically spell something out. I'd get frustrated and give up.

John's description of the embarrassment that frequently happens with this dyslexic learning style helped us understand why he avoided reading. The reaction of his classmates contributed to the panic and horror he experienced in reading in a group.

School was real frustrating. One time in English class in high school, we all had to read out loud. I had to read this passage and it was quite embarrassing because I misread, "brought the beast out in her." I said "brought the breast out of her." Everybody thought it was real funny, but it was extremely difficult for me to live that down. People probably forgot about it to a certain extent, but it builds up real barriers for you. You don't want to go across that ground after a while. You don't want to put yourself open to that kind of ridicule.

John had great difficulty focusing his attention on his reading. He found that he had to read information several times in order to make sense of it. He consistently lost his place as he was reading and found himself rereading a line or skipping several lines. Our first efforts with John helped him understand what he was doing.

Before when I was reading, it was like I wasn't recognizing the word the way it was. I was reading it so quickly with my eyes that to go back in memory to look at it... to say it, after I had read it quickly, I would forget the word and the recognition of what that word was wouldn't come to mind right away.
Sometimes I would pick up a word from a line below or a line above and intermix them. I was taking words out, getting

kind of a broad picture of what I was reading, not so much word for word. Maybe I was even going up and down looking at the words instead of across. I would get a broad sense of the sentence. And if several lines below, a word ended with "ty," I would add it onto the word I was reading.

Before class, before you had taught me how to put the mind's eye "on point," I had not realized that I'd never concentrated on certain things. If I wanted to concentrate, I would have to go into kind of a dazed state to eliminate a visualization, so that I could control my mind's eye. Otherwise, what I was seeing and imaging were in conflict. My attention would just start going off.

The Davis Orientation Mastery training was very helpful for John. In addition, he learned to use the neurological impress reading technique described in Part 2, Chapter 9, "Strategies That Work," *Neurological Impress Reading* (p. 150) and *Tapping Technique* (p. 152). It was this combination of techniques that allowed him to progress very rapidly in gaining control.

Once I learned to put myself on point, I could concentrate. The information I was picking up was making real sense. I could identify with the information, retain it much better. In some respects, I had a lot more mobility with what I wanted to do with the information. The biggest difference was I was comprehending what the sentence was trying to say, what the main point was. It was right there.

Individuals who experience difficulty in controlling their talented visualization abilities all report the same types of confusion. John's description sounded very similar to Scott's.

The imagery of the mind's eye is very powerful. In a lot of cases, you'd start reading something and you would have a certain amount of interest in it. And the mind's eye begins to pick up on it and goes off with it. The rest of the information after that point, once your mind's eye has picked up on it and taken that information and started transmitting the image in your mind, is not from the book. The imagery is dimensional and very strong. After that you would just be looking at words, but not reading anything. It is just so strong that your interest isn't there for what your eyes are bringing in.

It's very difficult for people to understand this experience. But it's like sitting there trying to read and having a television turned on next to you at full bore with something you are interested in on the program. It creates a conflict in what you are attending to.

With my focus point, I can discipline myself to stay with what I am reading. The true meaning of the information is much easier to get because I've cut down such a dramatically distracting item.

When John read silently, he moved so quickly that he was unable to keep pace with the meaning of the selection. John learned to recognize the words in phrases. Previously, all words just followed one another without any emphasis. When he began to experience the Phrasing technique described in Part 2, Chapter 9, "Strategies That Work" (p. 154), he began to understand which words were connected.

Once I had learned to control my attention, the information would come in much easier. Then we went through breaking the sentences into word groups. That was very beneficial in reading because before that I was going to fast through everything. My eyes used to move with incredible speed across the line of print. At first, it felt uncomfortable when I had to slow down. Getting things in "sync" was really uncomfortable.

Once we got into grouping the words and allowed the expression to flow into it, that gave it a real meaning. Before, the monotone was real boring. I think that as I started to get bored because it didn't sound right, I pulled myself off point. I learned to recognize what I was doing. I began to read just like I was breathing. Read to the end of a breath and then relax and start another group of words. It's just like talking.

Tapping out the punctuation helped a lot, too. It made me really aware of content. It's like someone turning the light up a bit. You know, the light starts out very dim in a room and you're trying to read and it's very difficult. If somebody turns the light up a little bit, well, it's a little bit easier and you realize this is better. What else can I do to increase the light to the point where it's really bright, so I can see and it's easy to read!

This part of the summer and the fall has been a real personal development part of my life. You know, there was a point in my life when reading wasn't really important. I doubt if I would have been so self-aware and so into learning. I think it's all relevant to certain people at certain times. It's really the right time for me.

A sense of control or power comes with the ability to focus attention. Our clients often felt that they didn't have the power to control their own thoughts or learning. When they experience control, they treasure the feeling. It tends to change their image of themselves. These are all very intelligent people. They have to be intelligent to support an active visualization and a creative thinking ability. Once they have learned to make their creative talents work for them, they open many choices in their lives which were previously closed to them.

Chapter Five

Dyslexia and Public Education

Each of the individuals who have shared their stories in this book were educated in our school systems. They may have attended school during different periods over the past twenty-five years, but their stories are remarkably similar. The unique needs of the dyslexic learning style have been overlooked or have been characterized as learning disabilities.

The incidence of reading problems in our society is astounding. While not all reading problems are caused by dyslexia, it is safe to speculate that some are dyslexic related. The impact of a major population of illiterates is of significant concern to our country.

APPALLING ILLITERACY

About a third of the people in the world over 15 years of age are illiterate. That is more than 815 million people. The dimensions of the problem are such that it qualifies as one of the great and continuing afflictions of mankind.

It is shocking to learn that illiteracy is also not only in our midst, but may be growing.

—San Francisco Chronicle, May 22, 1988, Editorials, R.T. Thieriot

We recognize that not all illiterates are dyslexic. There are many reasons for illiteracy. Lack of formal education, a different native language, vision or hearing handicaps, mental retardation, and a variety of other conditions may all contribute to illiteracy. No figures are available regarding the number of illiterates who cannot read because of dyslexia, but it is suspected that 10 to 15 percent of the population appear to have a mild to severe degree of dyslexia. Since the illiterate population is a specific subgroup of the regular population, one can expect that this select population will have an even higher level of dyslexics than the normal population.

Individuals like Annie, Richy, Jill, Carley, Scott, and John do not make national news when they announce that they have a dyslexic learning style. In the past five years, a number of publicly prominent individuals have admitted their frustration with reading and learning. These individuals receive tremendous publicity and their admission has provided public recognition that this unique learning style does exist.

The school histories they share will sound quite familiar when compared to those shared by our clients. The impact on their lives readily parallels that of the adults who have shared their stories. Because these individuals are important public figures , including movie stars and sports figures, their candor and openness may make a difference.

TOM CRUISE

Born Thomas Cruise Mapother IV on July 3, 1962 the third of four children and the only son he faced one barrier early on: dyslexia, the learning disability shared by an estimated 5 to 10 percent of all Americans and 4 to 7 percent of school-age children. "For me, it began in kindergarten," Cruise recalls. "I was forced to write with my right hand when I wanted to use my left. I began to reverse letters, and reading became so difficult. I was always ashamed, like we were the dummies."

Because his father traveled from job to job as an engineer, the family was constantly moving, and Cruise went to 15 different schools. "That made the problem worse," he says. "With my reading difficulties, I'd never catch up. But people would excuse me: 'He's the new kid. We'll just help him through this year.'" As a result, Cruise says, his dyslex-

ia was never "officially" diagnosed.

But Cruise's mother, who had studied to become a teacher of special education, recognized his symptoms and tutored him in methods designed to overcome the disability. " I had to train myself to focus my attention," Cruise explains. " I became very visual and learned how to create mental images in order to comprehend what I read."

What was most important, Cruise adds, was facing his disability head on: "My mother said, 'Look, you're dyslexic, so you'll just have to work harder at what others take for granted.' The motivation had to come from me. I was going into my junior year of high school, and I vowed, 'This time I won't be in the remedial class.' I worked very hard to bring my reading up to grade level so I could feel that I fit in."

—Parade Magazine, January 8, 1989, Ellen Hawkes

MANLEY'S SECRET SHAME: NFL STAR DESCRIBES PAIN OF ILLITERACY

Washington—Tearfully giving up on his written testimony, the Washington Redskins' Dexter Manley told a congressional committee yesterday how he played four years of college football and became all-pro without ever learning to read.

Under the hot glare of TV lights, sweat mingled with tears on Manley's face as he stumbled over his prepared statement to a Senate panel pondering national illiteracy. After the first paragraph, he stopped trying to read it.

"You're doing fine. This takes more courage than anything you've done on a football field," said Senator Paul Simon, D-Ill., as Manley struggled to regain his composure.

The packed hearing room was silent as Wally Amos, founder of the Famous Amos cookie chain and spokesman for the Literacy Volunteers of America, came to the witness table and comforted Manley, a 280-pound defensive end.

Then Manley told a Senate education subcommittee of his years of shame as a secret illiterate. He recalled how he pro-

gressed through a Houston high school and Oklahoma State University as a star athlete without every being expected to be a student, too.

"The only thing that made me feel good was athletic," he said. In the classroom, he "felt dumb and stupid," but "I was passed, of course."

At Oklahoma State, Manley stayed eligible to play football for four years but did not graduate.

"You didn't fail, sir. The system failed you," Senator Barbara Mikulski, D-Md., told Manley.

Simon, Chairman of the Senate Subcommittee on Education, Arts and Humanities, is sponsoring the Illiteracy Elimination Act of 1989. He told Manley that his reading problems are hardly unique.

"At least 23 million Americans lack the basic reading, writing and computational skills necessary to function effectively in our society," said Simon. The Illinois Senator said Manley's courage in admitting his problems and seeking help should inspire others to do likewise.

Manley, 30, who was paid over $400,000 by the Redskins last year, was the star witness in a hearing on "The Challenge of Eliminating Illiteracy." Since 1986, he has studied at the Lab School of Washington, where he was diagnosed as having a learning disability.

Sarah Hines, Manley's tutor at the Lab School, said he suffers from an "auditory channel" learning disability and has difficulty remembering words or sounding them out. The problem was never diagnosed during Manley's 17 years in school.

It has nothing to do with whether he is intelligent or not," she said.

Describing his education, Manley said he repeated the second grade and then was put into a special education class. "I felt I shouldn't be there," he said, describing his frustration and how he pushed his teacher against the blackboard.

But he stayed in the "special ed" class throughout elemen-

tary school. What he remembers from those years is "playing with blocks" and feeling inferior scholastically as he was taunted by schoolmates in regular classes.

"Kids are more cruel than anything else," he said.

By his junior high years though, Manley's athletic abilities were noticed and his classroom failures were overshadowed by success on the playing fields.

The push to end his illiteracy came on the sidelines of a Redskins game with the New York Giants in 1985, Manley said. Redskin quarterback Joe Theismann went down with a broken leg that eventually ended his football career.

Manley said he thought, "I hope this never happens to me; what would I do then?" without football. He heard about the Lab School and began his work there the next year.

—San Francisco Chronicle, May, 1989, Bob Dart

There are important similarities in the stories of our clients and these nationally prominent men. They received neither understanding or assistance from the educational system. Nor were they fortunate enough to find a teacher who was trained in working with individuals with dyslexic learning styles.

The impact of an illiterate population, which includes our dyslexic population, is of even greater concern when the individuals graduate from school and enter our job market. Today's jobs require reading skills as well as skills in organization, listening for directions, and writing. Many of the large corporations who have experienced this impact are asking for our schools to provide this missing education.

CAN YOUR WORKERS READ?

...As Motorola, Inc., Vice President Carlton Braun told the congressional Joint Economic Committee last April: "We have found to our disappointment that many workers are not prepared to operate the factory of the present, much less of the future."

Only 20 percent of job applicants at Motorola can pass a simple seventh grade test of English comprehension or a fifth grade mathematics test. New York Telephone Company reported that in a six month period of 1987, an astounding 84 percent of its job applicants failed the entry-level examination.

Behind those results are disturbing statistics such as these: Some 27 million adults are functionally illiterate, meaning they are unable to perform every day tasks such as writing a bank check, filling out a job application or identifying the deduction for Social Security on a wage statement. The ranks of the nation's functional illiterates grow each year by an estimated 2.3 million, including newcomers from abroad. In addition, some 40 million more adults are considered barely competent in those skills, and their number also is growing.

When estimates of both types of illiteracy are combined, it suggests that about 30 percent of adults about 1 our of 3 potential employees can't read, write or reason well enough to compete in today's economy.

—Nations' Business, October, 1988, Karen Berney

The impact of an illiterate population on our economy is staggering. It is equally overwhelming to our heavily burdened educational system. If the population of individuals with dyslexia were to be served through special education services, it would quickly overwhelm the system.

The majority of our school systems are not prepared to provide technically competent remediation programs which can enable dyslexic students to be successful in the regular classroom. The numbers of students eligible for special education services is increasing at an alarming rate; therefore, our regular education teachers need to learn techniques for teaching the individual with a dyslexic learning style. Once the unique learning style is understood, it is hoped that the adaptation of programs for group instruction and early preventive programs will become common practice in regular classrooms.

In the interim, our public school system is charged with providing special education services for students with learning disabilities. According to Public Law 94142, the Education for All Handicapped Children Act of 1975, students with dyslexia are included in the conditions described as learning disabilities. It reads:

> *"Specific learning disability" means a disorder in one or more of the basic psychological processes involved in understanding or using language, spoken or written, which may manifest itself in an imperfect ability to listen, think, speak, read, write, spell, or to do mathematical calculations. The term includes such conditions as perceptual handicaps, brain injury, minimal brain dysfunction, dyslexia, and developmental aphasia. The term does not include children who have learning problems which are primarily the result of visual, hearing or motor handicaps, of mental retardation, or of environmental, cultural, or economic disadvantages. (Section 5(b)(4) of P.L. 94142.)*

Dyslexia is specifically mentioned in this federal law. Several states have enacted legislation to specifically identify the dyslexic learner and some states provide specific programs to assist dyslexic students. Unfortunately, not all states have chosen to recognize this unique type of learning disability.

When a student is identified as eligible for special education, the programming provided usually addresses the specific content problem. For instance, students who are behind in reading receive more reading instruction, and those with spelling problems write their words more times or are given an easier list of words. In remediation programs, there is a definite trend to increased time-on-task and a breakdown of the task into smaller increments for learning. Students are still being provided with flash cards and other systems which have questionable worth for dyslexic students.

The case studies in this book show that with identification and training, individuals with a dyslexic learning style can function successfully in regular programs. The goal we have for these students is to be effective, efficient learners. They do not have to fight their way through the school system and hide from reading. Their parents should not have to suffer and be humiliated in order to find an education for their children.

Three Phases of Learning

Basic Processing Skills	Strategies	Academic Skills

Memory Skills
  Visual
    Auditory
    Motor
 	
Attention Focus
    Time Senses
    Stimulus Filter
 	
Motor
Coordination
    Balance
 	
Rhythm
 	
Language
	Visualization
	
	Re-verbalization
	
	Integration
	
	Study Skills
		Reading
		
		Comprehension
		
		Spelling
		
		Writing Skills
		
		Math

Chapter Six

You Can Do It!
Success Stories

In 1968, Melvin-Smith Learning Center began working with cognitive therapy programs for clients with head trauma (brain injury). These individuals experienced specific injuries and associated loss of cognitive processing skills. By working with them, we learned that no one area of our brain has sole responsibility for the complex functions required for speaking, reading, writing and reasoning. Each skill requires a "chaining" or interconnectedness of active and supportive areas. When the sequence was interrupted because of a brain injury, the cognitive skill requiring the support of these areas became partially or completely interrupted.

We designed cognitive therapy programs which required the client to simulate the desired activity or skill. Initially we broke the skill down, isolating all the necessary components within a complex hierarchy. We then began the therapy with tasks which approximated each step in the chain. With the success of each step, the individual came nearer to performing the skill. The skills became part of the individual's repertoire of abilities. The changes were readily observed and could be measured objectively through intellectual assessments.

The three level intervention system (processing, strategies and academic skills) is used to establish the actual programming activities.

THREE PHASES OF LEARNING
Processing:
Identification and training of processing skills which are

needed for strengthening memory, perception, attention, tracking and/ or language.

Strategies:

Application of visualization techniques, reverbalization, study skills (mind mapping, charting, outlining, note taking), and logic and reasoning. These techniques teach the individual to use their processing skills and talents for academic or work related applications.

Academic Skills:

Emphasis is on basic academic skills such as reading, writing, spelling and math. An important element is the selection of a reading and spelling system which will be successful. It is very important to understand that different reading systems are effective depending upon the age, learning profile, and experience of the individual prior to training.

The effectiveness of our system is in the training of the support skills which the brain uses in order to store and recall information effectively. This is why emphasis is placed on the processing and strategies portion of the training program. Once the brain is prepared to learn, the acquisition of academic information is quite comfortable and a reading/spelling system from a broad range of choices can be successful. If the brain is not prepared for learning, most reading/spelling systems will not be effective because the individual can not receive or retain information accurately and in the quantity needed for success in reading. Since most of our clients are anxious for rapid progress in their reading/spelling skills, it is essential to work on all three intervention levels simultaneously.

The emotion that accompanies success for individuals with dyslexic learning styles is joy. It often includes the release of tears for the many years of frustration, the posture that radiates success and confidence and the smile that says *"I can't believe it, but I did it!"* It is time to celebrate. Included within this final chapter of Part One, are success stories to provide hope and the knowledge that success in academic skill development is possible.

ANNIE

Annie experienced visual symbol confusion. Her intelligence enabled her to evade reading for a long period of time. She could not recall the word images and mis-sequenced her letters. Our programming for Annie included the following:

Processing:
1. Visual sequential memory training
2. Directional training and spatial organization

Strategies:
1. Learning to utilize visualization skills for improving visual symbol memory
2. Goal setting to include "I can read."

Academics:
1. Easing Into Reading for reading and spelling.
2. Auditory Discrimination in Depth for reading.
3. Neurological Impress spelling.

As symbols began to appear familiar to Annie, she found that she could recognize words and she began to write. She relaxed her fear of failing and became quite amused with the process of reading. Her mother observes this change:

> *Every year since she was born, Annie's grandmother, a kindergarten teacher, had brought her books. Each time they would sit down to enjoy the books, Annie would tell her grandmother that she enjoyed listening to them. She would listen to her grandmother read for as long as possible. However, if it*

was suggested that Annie read to her grandmother she was visibly upset and refused to participate any longer.

For Christmas this year, one year after Annie began her training program, Annie bought a book for her grandmother for Christmas. The card on the gift read:

Grandma, I will read this one to you.

Love, Annie

The phonetic approach was very successful for Annie. It provided her with a system upon which she could base her decisions for attacking a new word. Previous to this, she had memorized words from a specific story, but could not recognize the word if it were out of context.

Her strong intellectual abilities complicated her remediation. She had developed many compensatory and avoidance techniques to keep her away from reading and from being discovered. As she developed memory skills for symbols and learned to use her visualization talents for symbol recall, she began to risk learning a symbol system.

Goal setting was very important for Annie because it allowed her to identify the small steps which would enable her to reach her goal of being a good reader. Some of the goal statements we set with Annie included: *"I will be able to repeat four symbols from memory after a five second observation." "I will tell myself I am a real reader four times each day,"* and *"I will recognize the 'b' symbol each time I see it."* Annie's instructor writes about her progress:

She has worked hard and has taken great pride in her accomplishments. She has shown good growth in her ability to decode words and uses a variety of skills (context clues, pictures, predicting, etc.) to increase her reading ability. Annie's vivid imagination and love for fantasy have certainly motivated her in both her reading and writing. When she wants to hear a story or tell one, she reads and writes almost effortlessly.

Annie is learning to evaluate her writing in terms of whether it conveys what she originally intended. Work with spelling, punctuation and reading are emphasized in a variety of activities to achieve this goal. Making detailed and correct mental maps of visual images is also being used to help her to record information correctly.

Annie responded positively to the challenge of doing activities she once thought too difficult. Her hard work has resulted in increased self-esteem and pride. A weekly record in which she records her feelings towards school and reading, reflects that she has positive feelings about both. She rates them a seven on a scale from one to ten.

Annie was reassessed in November after several months of intensive programming. As a third grader, she scored a 3.1 (third grade, first month) grade level score and a 92 Standard Score. Her reading comprehension scored at 6.8 grade level with a Standard Score of 123. She recognizes that she can read, and with continued intervention her reading skills will be able to support her exceptional intellectual level.

RICHY

Richy was twenty-nine when we first met him. The story he shared in the opening chapter and again in the Visual Symbol Confusion (Chapter Two) moved all of us at the Melvin-Smith Learning Center. We were as committed to teaching him to read as he was determined to read.

Richy was very motivated to be successful in reading. He could not recognize basic symbols consistently and the sequencing of the symbols was constantly changing for him. His program focused on the following areas:

Processing:
  1. Orientation Counseling

2. Development of visual symbol memory skills from single digit to six digit recall
3. Development of auditory memory skills from three digit to seven digit recall

Strategies:
1. Awareness of language transformations and familiarity with written grammar consistencies
2. Visualization strategies for imaging words and recalling them for spelling

Academics:
1. The Auditory Phonics Program (TAPP) for reading and spelling
2. Auditory Discrimination in Depth (ADD) program for reading

Richy learned to use the multi/kinesthetic technique of his reading programs to figure out his words. However, he continued to experience an inability to automatically recognize the words until he had advanced his visual sequential memory to five digits. At that point, he started to recognize familiar letter groups as words and began to build his automatic vocabulary.

He is now being successful. He has gained three years in reading. Most important to us, he has increased his ability to recall visually represented symbols. His memory skills have moved from below the charts into the average range. This means that he will increase in his learning speed and his long term recall can grow even more rapidly. He can continue to add new words to his reading and spelling vocabulary just by experiencing them as he reads.

Richy spent twenty-two years failing in learning. He has spent sixteen months succeeding. In his most recent testing, he saw that his scores were really changing and he was learning. His smile beamed across the room. He wanted to share this information with others. The dialogue between Richy and his Clinician reflects his feelings.

Clinician: *We just finished the retesting on you and it is so exciting to see what has happened to you over the course of your programming. You are reading now and your scores have gone up three years. You are reading words that are multi-syllable words; that are difficult words to read. You are spelling words phonetically. How do you feel about what is happening?*

Richy: *Well, the only word I can find is wonderful! I feel wonderful 'cause I can read things I could never read before in my life. It's helping me to understand things. For one, I can read the Bible. Something I never could do, but wanted to do. I can find my way around on a map, something I never could do. And I can handle myself better on the job. I'm not great at it yet, but I am planning on getting there. And just knowing that in a year, it's been a year, that I have started to pick it up. Just knowing that I can really read has changed my life.*

I feel more alert and more positive about myself. I feel like I can really challenge the world now and it's something I don't want to stop because it's like the doors are really open for me now. I really want to challenge everything. I want to learn a whole lot more because now I see what I have been missing. I knew that I was missing a lot, but I really didn't know how much. But now I do. It makes you really want to try harder 'cause you learn more and more and it's so exciting every time you make one step further. It's like the sun is shining in your heart.

I knew how important reading was, but just knowing how important it was for me didn't make it happen. Now I can do it and I don't feel unhappy any more. I can sit and take a book by myself and read without asking someone to read the book to me. If I make a mistake, I can go to the sounds and figure it out myself and it is right.

Clinician: *Is there anything you want to share? I know you have had a lot of changes in your life. You are working now and you have just gotten engaged.*

Richy: *I have a positive frame of mind now. I feel more relaxed. You know, I feel like I have a chance. When I couldn't read, I didn't think I had a chance in the world. But now with the Learning Center, you and Dr. Smith, you understand me. You have trust in me that I can do it. Thank the Lord that it did happen. It's kind of like I have power in myself.*

I was thinking just the other day, how much I really want to put back. Because I know there are a lot of other people, women and men, that can't read. By me knowing what I went through and what I am experiencing now, if I can be a teacher someday, even just help one person, then I feel that I would put something back. And that person might help somebody else. That's what I really want to do, but I have a long way to go yet. I just really thank you and Dr. Smith for all you have done. I hope I can just make you guys proud, because I am.

Clinician: *I just want to say how rewarding it has been to work with you. You have been so motivated and your desire to read has been so great. To see you read and to hear you read has been such a pleasure.*

Richy: *For you to hear me read! It's a thrill to hear myself read. I laugh about it sometimes. I say, "Did I say this did I read this? Did I read this whole book?" And I throw the book in the air and I catch it, and I say, "I did it!"*

I really think its going to make me go further. I am sure it's going to make me go further and the more I go to school, the more I learn and the more I am going to challenge.

As far as my work, I can buy a tool like a paint gun. I bought one and I really sat down and read the directions. I read it and I used it. Something I could have never done before. I always had to figure it out before. Of course, it taught me because once I figured it out I never forgot it. Now it's easier because I can read it, figure it out and do it. Something that would have taken me two hours to do before, now takes me thirty minutes. It saves a lot of time now that I can read.

Even on the job, if I go out and do a little work, I can write out a bill now. I don't have to go home and have somebody write it up for me. Now I can write it up and sign it and give it to the customer. It's going to help a lot. It really is.

All I can say to other people is don't give up. 'Cause all of those fifteen years, I never gave up. It took a lot of looking and trying, but I never gave up. And this is my reward, even if it took a long time. I never gave up and I hope others don't give up because it can happen for them. Just don't give up, it will happen!

This dialogue from Richy is especially important because it reflects his growth, not just in reading, but in language. The dialogue in the beginning of the book included classic grammatical errors which are frequently observed with individuals with a dyslexic learning style. His programming included work on language and the transformations in grammar. Now that his listening skills have improved and he is reading, his language has changed significantly.

CARLEY

Carley completed her training program during the summer. She was unable to receive tutoring during the school year because of transportation problems. Her mother attempted to arrange a three-week intensive program during the past fall for Carley so that she could rescue what was becoming another frustrating school year. It seemed that Carley was continuing to be late for class, miss assignments and be discouraged. The school was phoning frequently to complain about her lack of study skills.

An intensive program could not be arranged for Carley because one of her subject teachers said that if she missed three weeks of classes, he would not pass her. The school did not recognize her learning challenges and her unique dyslexic learning style. Nor could it be flexible in providing her the opportunity to change it.

This summer Carley completed her intensive programming. It was an exciting adventure for her. Her programming emphasized the following areas:

Processing:
1. Auditory memory and listening skills development
2. Rhythm development
3. Attention focus training

Strategies:
1. Language transformations and vocabulary development (analogies programming)
2. Time and space organization
3. Study skills
4. Synchronization of visual/auditory processing for reading (neurological impress reading with tapping and phrasing)

Academics:
1. Comprehension
2. Neurological Impress Reading
3. Neurological Impress Spelling

This program provided a full menu for Carley. She was well motivated to be a good student since she wanted to attend college and needed to obtain the grades for admission. Her processing skills began to develop quite quickly as she understood the need to use all of her brain resources for success. The emphasis on understanding time and organization was quite important for Carley. She worked on setting up a daily schedule and began to anticipate the amount of time it would take to accomplish different tasks. She learned to make a list of everything she needed to do and to check it off as she accomplished her tasks. She was very pleased with herself as she found this system working.

She took on several jobs during her training time, including planning a luncheon in great detail. She used the who, where, what, when, how, and why planning to guide herself. She transferred this to her planning for school. She developed her own checklist for getting better grades at school. It included: *1. Do your homework. 2. Go to class. 3. Be on time. 4. Limit your talking while the teacher is lecturing, during tests and during quiet study times. 5. Talk to the teachers and let them know your goals and request their help.*

Understanding time and organization was critical for Carley in view of her school history. She was unable to organize herself in school and could not follow through on her intentions. Now she has practiced and found that she can turn her intentions into actions and can schedule herself.

In addition, Carley has developed a system for understanding what she is reading. She understands the rhythm and phrasing of language. She can comprehend what she is reading when she synchronizes the word she is looking at and the word she is saying. Tapping is used to assist her in gaining synchronized understanding.

Phonics instruction assisted her in understanding the syllables and sounds in spelling. She found that she could utilize the training to rapidly enlarge her writing vocabulary. She will be continuing to fine tune her skills during the school year. For the first time in nine years, Carley is looking forward to school starting. She is organized and prepared for success.

JILL

Last summer made the difference for Jill. At the age of fifteen, she was being recommended for dismissal from special education services because of lack of cooperation. Despite the special education support, she received failing grades in language and math. She was the only girl in the program and was constantly teased about being in special education. Jill was terrified at the prospect of being removed from the program where she had been safe since mid-elementary years. At the same time, she did not feel that she was learning any new skills. She felt like she was just sitting there and being bored. She was being uncooperative because of her feelings of failure.

Just before school started Jill participated in an intensive program. The activities included the following emphasis:

Processing:
  1. Attention training (balance beam and eye contact emphasis)
  2. Rhythm skills

Strategies:
  1. Synchronization of visual/auditory processing (neurological impress reading)
  2. Study Skills (mind mapping for composition development and note taking)

Academics:
  1. Comprehension development
  2. Spelling—Neurological Impress
  3. Word Attack—Educators Publishing Co.

During her summer programming, Jill learned that she could be successful. First she had to learn to control her attention focus. Jill was very powerful in creative imagery. When she diverted her attention, it was frequently to image something she was thinking about. Her eyes would immediately shift into a visual accessing position, (upward and off to the side), and she would not be listening. It was this urge to alter her attention focus from the speaker that Jill needed to learn to control.

She learned to recognize when her attention would stray by using the attention training program on the balance beam. She increased her attention focus and learned to resist diverting it. When she could maintain her focus for five minutes, she had resisted her tendency to disorient at least ten times. This was sufficient to give her the control over her attention.

She began to understand how to use her visual strengths for retaining spelling words. She practiced imaging the words and storing them for later access. She used the Word Attack program by Josephine Rudd (Educator's Publishing Company) for a review of syllabication and phonic development.

By the end of her three week intensive program, her test scores in reading, spelling, vocabulary, and general knowledge had increased between two and three years. Jill was still scheduled to return to special education and was terrified to think about leaving special class and being in a regular classroom.

We evaluated Jill's skills and recommended to her that she participate in the regular program. On two occasions, Jill brought a friend to her staffing review and on both occasions her friends encouraged her to be in the regular program with them.

We were concerned about the lack of expectations in continuing in special class where Jill had three periods each day. When she entered the class, the teacher would have a sentence on the board which the students were to copy and correct. Then they were to work on their regular class work with the help of the special education teacher and aide. She received no direct instruction for learning a spelling system, no comprehension training, and no study skills assistance. The program would best be described as "homework support."

Despite our best efforts to convince Jill that she was ready to leave special education, she chose to continue for one more semester. She agreed that she would make the transition in

January. We felt it was important that she make this choice herself and promised to abide by her decision.

At this point, it appears that the fates intervened. The school computer scheduled her in college prep classes with no special education. The special education teacher was horrified and said she couldn't possibly handle regular classes. Her mother was upset and while everyone scrambled around to have the schedule changed, Jill decided that she liked being in the regular classes. By the end of her first day in school, she decided to stay in her new program.

Jill worked for several hours each night to keep up with her new studies. She was supported by a tutor, who had received training at the Learning Center as part of Jill's intensive, to carry on with Jill's programming. She used her time with her tutor very effectively. She achieved all A's and B's on her report card. She even received an A in Reading class from a teacher that had seen her as a "problem" the previous year. All of her citizenship grades were Excellent and Satisfactory. One teacher wrote, *"Jill has really improved this year. She has a whole new attitude and it shows in her work! She's going to do just great!"* The math teacher wrote, *"Great first quarter in math!"*

Jill will be coming to spend a few weeks with us again this summer. She has already informed us of her goals: to work on her spelling and comprehension. She wants to get ready for high school next year so she *"can keep her grades up for college."*

Our clients who experience the Attention Focus learning style can move the most rapidly of all. Jill showed the difference it made when she learned to control her attention. Scott experienced the same changes at the age of thirty-five.

SCOTT

Scott spent several months with a two hour a week training program to develop his attention skills and learn a reading system. During this time, he went from failing at his computerized accounting program to teaching the class. He has since been fully employed in his new field and continues to be successful with his skills.

The programming activities which were most important for Scott included the following:

Processing:
    1. Attention focus Orientation Counseling

Strategies:
    1. Synchronization of visual auditory processing
    2. Logic and reasoning skills.

Academics:
    1. Comprehension: Neurological Impress Reading
    2. The Auditory Phonics Program: reading/spelling
    3. Auditory Discrimination in Depth

A major change in his abilities to process occurred for Scott immediately following the Orientation Counseling. He began to be able to screen out distractions from his environment and to focus his attention with great success. This allowed him to use the reading skills he was gaining through the phonics programs. He reported his success as follows:

> *You know in just six months, I have got the urge to read. I just noticed it a few days ago. I was sitting down to eat breakfast cereal and all of a sudden I am reading all four sides of the box, top and bottom! Before I wouldn't even have thought about it. I'm having a pretty good time with it. Things seem to be better.*

In addition to his improved reading skills, he recognized his ability to stay focused. The orientation counseling which improved his attention focus training was referenced in these comments.

I can still visualize anytime I want to. But before the problem was I couldn't control it. Now I can and I can keep things from distracting me. Before, when people were saying things, I could feel myself start to drift off. I would drift off and then gradually come back and miss a bunch of stuff. Now I can feel myself drifting off and when I do that, I put myself right back on point and it happens so fast that I never miss any information.

I found out that I don't get so irritable anymore. I used to get mad. It's like I would be doing something and the kids would go by or say something or make noise and I would be mad. They would interrupt me and I would have to go back and start over from the beginning. Now I can shut them out of my mind. I can keep working and it doesn't bother me.

Two things have really changed for me. I used to be sitting in class reading something and yet I was listening to everyone talking. I'd get real mad because it bothered me. Now I have learned to deal with it because I can keep reading and ignore everything and not even hear it. And the other thing is, I understand what I am reading.

Scott's growth enabled him to find a position in his new field. In each of the areas he had feared failing, he was now successful.

JOHN
John experienced the same success at age thirty-five. He found that he could maintain his attention and not be distracted by his highly developed visualization system. John's programming included the following areas of concentration:

Processing:
1. Attention focus Orientation Counseling
2. Rhythm

Strategies:
1. Synchronization of visual/auditory processing (neurological impress reading with tapping and phrasing)

Academics:

1. Comprehension: Neurological Impress Reading

John learned to control his attention skills. He found that he could process conversations without being distracted. The Davis Orientation Counseling was very helpful for John. It quickly provided him with a means of centering his attention and controlling his visualization talents.

His reading improved from the training in learning to synchronize his visual and auditory systems as he was reading. It radically and quickly changed his comprehension ability. His comprehension score moved from below average to above average. His spelling score moved from a Standard Score of 75 to 90 in twenty-one hours of instruction.

> *I'd never concentrated on certain things before my classes. I never realized how much I missed. If I had concentrated, I would have to go into a kind of a dazed state to eliminate visualization, so that I could use nothing but my mind's eye to visualize. There was a conflict between the two. My eyes and my mind's eye would give me different information. I'd get two real strong conflicting sets of information. And then the two, you know, sometimes it's a real battle which is the stronger. Sometimes the mind's eye would have the strong hand and actually put the concentration right out.*
>
> *So I would just start to go off and lose my attention to what was going on in front of me. But once I learned to stay on point, I could control it. The information I saw was really making a lot more sense. I gained the choice about what I wanted to do with the information. I understood it and I could make use of it. I was in control.*

It is this feeling of control that the individual with a dyslexic learning style treasures when he or she finally experiences it. It is being able to listen and make sense of something that is said. It is reading a paragraph and remembering what it is about. It is being able to plan and organize thoughts, papers, and environment. It is being able to find a place on a map or follow a direction. For each of these individuals, gaining control of his or her mind means success.

Individuals who experience the unique learning style of the dyslexic can be successful in reading, comprehending, spelling and improving their attention skills. The individuals who have shared their stories in this book are living proof of the success that can be gained. Representing a wide variety of ages, profiles and opportunities, they all have two important elements in common. They have experienced the frustration of a dyslexic learning style and they have experienced the success of finding that they do not have to be dyslexic.

You Don't Have To Be Dyslexic

PART TWO

Remediation For Success

Chapter Seven

Evaluating the Learning Style

When children enter school they begin their experiences with letters, words and numbers as the beginning steps for reading and math. Some children's brains are ready to begin recalling symbols and sequencing symbolic information when they enter school, while others are not. Our experience at the Melvin-Smith Learning Center is that students with a dyslexic learning style can be identified at this time by their lack of readiness in processing skills.

Our most common error in education is assuming that the child is ready for learning when he or she enters kindergarten. We refer to this as a Type One Error. The second most common error, Type Two Error, is recognizing that the child is not ready and assuming that it is because they are "immature."

An assumption prevails that children come to school with the necessary visual and auditory memory skills to recall symbols and to sequence sounds. It is assumed that the student perceives the symbols accurately and that the symbols hold still and look the same each time they are seen. It is assumed that the student has adequate attention skills and has an understanding of the passage of time. And it is assumed that the student is ready to learn to organize the complex system of reading and writing. The error in this assumption is that we do not recognize what the student is experiencing. We miss the fact that their processing systems are not "on" or ready. Reading instruction begins, and students begin to fail through no fault or control of their own.

Scenario: *The Type One child enters school with skills which* *suggest that they can learn. When they begin to receive reading (symbol) instruction, they exhibit signs of stress and confusion. The highly intelligent child may figure out temporary ways of coping, like Annie (Chapter Two), who memorized what she heard and could pretend to read by repeating what she recalled. Assuming that since she appeared intelligent she would have the necessary skills to begin reading, the school did not notice her reading disability. It was her mother who was alerted to the problem by Annie's mounting stress.*

The Type Two Error manifests itself when an educator recognizes that the student is not ready and labels the lack of readiness as "immaturity." Webster's New World Dictionary defines "immature" as "not mature; not completely developed" and "not finished or perfected."

Scenario: The Type Two kindergarten student comes to school along with his age mates. The teacher observes that he does not want to color, has trouble staying in his seat, seems wiggly during story time and becomes frustrated with structured tasks. The teacher identifies him as immature and recommends that he stay home or in preschool programs where he can "mature" for another year.

Even first and second grade students are retained in a grade so that they can "mature." The implication in our educational community is that time or aging will solve the problem. Aging is not usually a solution when the problem is a lack of development of processing skills. Interventions are needed to correct the problem. In fact, the passive approach of waiting is detrimental to the child's progress, self esteem and feelings of competency. It is essential to conduct an assessment to accurately understand the individual's learning profile.

ASSESSMENT

The purpose of an assessment is to identify how an individual is learning. To know where the interventions are needed, we must identify the individual's learning skills. The questions that should be answered by an assessment include each of the areas identified as learning attributes. The issues covered by an assessment include:

PROCESSING
Memory for Symbols
1. How much information (number of items including numerals, letters, words or sentences) can the individual remember when he HEARS and has to REPEAT the information from memory?
2. How much information can the individual remember when he HEARS and has to WRITE the information from memory?
3. How much information can the individual remember when he SEES and has to REPEAT the information from memory?
4. How much information can the individual remember when he SEES and has to WRITE the information from memory?

This part of the assessment will provide both memory skill and channel preference information. From this information, the assessor will be able to evaluate perceptual and spatial organization skills. Rotations of letters and errors in sequencing will be readily apparent, as will the amount of information (digit span) which the individual can recall. Suggested assessment instruments include: Receptive Expressive Observation, Detroit Test of Learning Aptitudes, Slingerland, and others which provide memory information.

PROCESSING
Memory for pictures
5. How many items can the individual recall when pictures are used instead of symbols (words or letters)?

An essential issue in looking at the visual processing skills is the differentiation between recall of concrete or pictorial information compared to symbolic information. Many students with the visual talent observed in dyslexia are exceptional in recalling pictures or experiences. Suggested assessments instruments include: Detroit Test of Learning Aptitudes and teacher/specialist made tests.

PROCESSING
Attention
6. How long can the individual maintain attention on a learning (or testing) task and what is likely to distract them?
   A. Observe and document length of attention focus at the beginning of an hour of assessment versus length of attention at the end.
   B. Observe and identify distracters and the stimuli that create distractions: environmental sounds, visual items in the environment, their own body (hair, nails, clothing) or their own internal thoughts.
   C. Ask the individual to walk , heel to toe, forward and backward on a line while maintaining eye contact with a target on the wall (placed at eye level. Use a stop watch to time the attention focus. Stop after two minutes or when she averts her eyes from the target.
7. Does the individual provide eye contact with the assessor and where do the eyes focus when he is seeking an answer?

This component is important for identifying the degree to which attention focus will create an interference in learning. Observations of eye movement patterns may provide information regarding the particular memory system that is in use. These observations can be made during any of the academic or memory assessments.

PROCESSING
Rhythm
8. Can the individual retain a rhythm pattern and repeat it for a one minute period?

This is another informal evaluation task in which the ability to internalize rhythms is observed. Rhythms are important in reading and are utilized in our remediation program, so it is important to evaluate this skill.

PROCESSING
Language
9. Does the individual appear to have good language skills including vocabulary, adequate length of sentences, and use of a variety of sentence patterns?

Language assessments are usually available through speech and language pathologists and educational psychologists. Information can be gained informally, however, by a good listener. Listen for compute verbalizations, noun/verb agreement, correct pronunciation of words and accurate labeling.

ACADEMIC SKILLS
Reading, Spelling and Math
10. What are the reading/spelling skills the individual is presently demonstrating?

Observations of error patterns may provide indicators of specific academic challenges which can be formally evaluated. Suggested assessment instruments which allow observation of the client working include: Wide Range Achievement Test Spelling subtest, Peabody Individual Achievement Test Reading Recognition and Reading Comprehension subtests, Boder Test of Reading and Spelling, Kaufman Test of Educational

Achievement, Kaufman Assessment Battery for Children, and Woodcock Johnson Psycho/Educational Battery.

INTERVIEWING

In addition to the formal assessment, it is essential to learn about the individual through an interview. The following series of questions can guide the discussion to discover talents and inefficiencies in learning:

Interviewing Questions:
1. What part of your day at school (work) is most comfortable for you? Listen for preferences and activities which reflect specific skills. For instance: the answer *"baseball"* presupposes athletic skills, *"being with the people at work"* suggests social skills and so on.

2. What is your least favorite activity/experience during the day? Identify indicators of areas which provide discomfort. For instance, if at work, entering the payroll on the computer leads to complaints about reversing numbers, visual memory inefficiencies may be apparent. If people taking a break and talking near the individual's desk are reported as disruptive, then maintaining attention with auditory interference could be an issue.
3. What is happening with your reading at this time? Children may report what reading group they are in or give situational descriptions, but what you want them to tell you is *how* are they trying to read. They may need to be prompted with questions such as:
    A. Do you use sounds to figure out a word or do you   recognize the way it looks?
    B. How do you try to figure out a word you haven't seen before?

Adults can be more specific than children. They will describe their frustrations with reading. They can identify if they experience dissynchrony between the word they are looking at and the one they are saying. They may relate that they read a sentence or a paragraph and have no idea what they have just read, although they may know in detail what is going on around them.

4. How do you spell a word you do not know? Their strategy for spelling words will be important information. Note the steps and processes used. If they describe shutting their eyes and trying to imagine the word, their spelling strategy is likely to be one of visual recognition. If they describe sounding out the letters in the word, they are attempting to use an auditory approach.

5. Ask about the memory testing that was done during the assessment.

   A. How did you remember when you saw the information?

   B. How did you remember when you heard it?

   C. Which felt easier?

   D. Was it easier to say it back or write it?

   Understanding the strategies used for remembering unrelated information is essential. Some may describe looking at the series of numbers, projecting them on the wall and reading them back from the projected image; others may repeat them silently over and over and finally say them out loud. Whatever the strategy, it reveals much about how efficiently their memory skills are being used.

6. Are there any other things you have experienced in reading or learning that would help me in understanding your skills? This question invites a sharing of the uniqueness of the individual's experiences in reading. Some will describe how the words seem to run off the page (disorientation) or how they get lost in the transi-

tion from one line to another (tracking). Individuals may tell of an incident in school where someone in authority told them they were stupid and would never learn to read. They may speak of the agony of not being able to read and the continual embarrassment. This is all important information for understanding the impact of being dyslexic on this individual's life.

The information to be gained from assessment and interviewing is essential in developing the program plan. It provides the direction and the insight to each individual's unique learning style. It is important for identifying the processing channels which require assistance, designing strategies, and selecting reading and spelling programs that will be effective.

Chapter Eight

Preparing the Brain for Learning

Processing skills must work efficiently to support learning. In order to adequately prepare the brain for learning, we evaluate the first phase of learning: **Processing** (memory, attention, rhythm and spatial organization). These are the skills which must in place for the brain to receive, comprehend, retain and retrieve symbolic information accurately.

In 1971, a young man of nineteen was sitting in the Learning Center office with his mother. We had just completed a diagnostic assessment for him. He was a nonreader and numerous attempts to teach him to read had been unsuccessful. He could not consistently recognize letter symbols and could only read a few words.

In our conversation with his mother, we were discussing visual memory. We had explained to both of them that one of the necessary activities the brain performed for us in reading was retaining visual symbols. We talked about being able to visualize a letter or a word. We explained to them that he appeared to have difficulty with his visual memory. We used the example of knowing what the word "cat" looked like. His mother said, *"Yes, I can shut my eyes and see how it is spelled."* At this point the young man leaned over with obvious concern for his mother and said, *"Mom, she's going to think you are crazy. Don't talk about seeing words in your head!"*

At nineteen, this student had never been aware of the visualization process. He had not developed a memory bank for words. He had not learned to use his visual memory to storage symbolic information. The topic which we were discussing must have appeared quite alien to him.

It was this client who initially prompted us to develop processing training. His observations about his lack of ability to visualize information caused us to begin to talk about "inner language." Throughout the seventies, we worked on developing an understanding of the types of inner language skills which were required for learning efficiently. The initial efforts focused on memory development.

Through our efforts with individuals with unique learning styles, we learned that the ability to accurately storage and efficiently access both visual and auditory memory is essential for skilled reading. While it sounds quite obvious, it is still a concept which is frequently challenged in the literature.

We firmly believe that when individuals are operating at a two or three unit (digit) visual and auditory memory level, they cannot retain reading and spelling vocabulary words. When they experience errors in either their visual or auditory memory, they experience inefficiencies in their reading and effective performance. Therefore, it is essential to prepare the brain for learning if we are going be successful in developing reading, comprehending and writing skills.

Annie, who was described in the **Visual Symbol Confusion** illustration, experienced visual memory confusion. She could not recall more than three letters. When she attempted to verbalize what she had just seen, she would forget parts of the sequence. When she saw *"b r g l,"* she would repeat *"d g r."*

During this same time period, Annie was being taught to read at school using flash cards. Every night the flash cards would be reviewed with her mother. During the day, the special reading teacher started each reading period with the flash cards. Sometimes Annie would know the word during the day and forget it that night. Sometimes she could not recall it at all. There was never any consistency. If they stopped working with the flash cards for a few days, she would forget all of them. Her visual memory could not support the task of imaging and recalling four to six letter units of information.

We had to teach Annie how to use her brain to remember. The first step was to identify what she was doing to remember. Annie had good language skills and strong verbal recall. We were suspicious that she was using her auditory memory to support learning. This was an accurate observation. Annie reported:

> *When I look at the word, I try to say the letters over and over again. Then I try to say the sounds of the letters real fast and sometimes the word just comes to me. It never really looks familiar, I have to figure it out every time from the letters and sounds.*

This was her system for attempting to read. She was being taught by a visual approach. She was attempting to convert the flash cards into an auditory approach by using her strength, her memory for sounds. This was not an efficient system for Annie and she could not perform consistently. While her teachers thought that she was remembering the words, she was actually furtively attempting to figure them out each time.

There are four processing skills (memory, attention, language and spatial organization) which can be taught and will prepare the brain for efficient learning. At the Melvin-Smith Learning Center, when a client is identified as having difficulty in any of these areas of processing, a program is established to develop these skills.

The activities for training in each of these skills for learners are provided in this chapter. Programming may be implemented in any setting: preschool programs, elementary classrooms, study skills courses, special education and/or tutoring settings for children or adult learners. They are essential in preparing the brain for learning and provide the basis for facilitating success.

The content and materials need to be adapted to the age and level of the individual; however, the patterns, systems and strategies are the same for all ages. They will successfully prepare the brain for learning.

PROCESSING STRATEGIES

The ability to storage information for later retrieval, memory, is one of the brain's most important functions. When memory problems are identified, we include specific training in the program plan. The training should take five to ten minutes during each session and should be done at least twice each week.

Both **visual** and **auditory** memory processing skills respond to training. Efficient access to memory facilitates learning and effective reading and spelling. Wc find that these skills impact on retention for the individual with a dyslexic learning style.

VISUAL MEMORY DEVELOPMENT

Visual symbol memory is a learned skill. Fortunately, most people develop visual memory skills very early, and subsequently are ready for symbol retention when they are between the ages of four and seven. If symbol recall is not learned, is inefficient, or for some reason is not used by the learner, then it will likely create serious reading/spelling dysfunction.

The elements of visual memory include:
Quantity: The amount of information or number of items to be retained. (Four letters, four numerals, four words, etc.)
Complexity: The type of information to be retained. For instance shapes are usually easier to recall than letters, numerals are easier than letters, letters are easier than words.

As an example, Annie could recall three items visually. When she attempted to retain four symbols, she would forget some or mix them. The quantity for Annie was three items. The complexity did not appear to stress her. She could retain three numerals, letters or shapes. She usually recalled the first items she saw correctly.

The individual who recalls the first of the information tends to rely on primacy. In other words the initial items seen are recalled, but later items are forgotten. It appears as though there are a certain number of memory spaces and when that is filled the rest is ignored. The pattern will appear as follows:

Primacy Example:

Stimulus	Response
2 3 4 5 6	2 3 4
b r t y w	b r t
cat, run, hat	cat, run

Other individuals will rely on recency. This means that they will recall the most recent item seen. Their response pattern will look like this:

Recency Example:

Stimulus	Response
2 3 4 5 6	5 6
b r t y w	t y w
cat, run, hat	hat

Understanding how Annie was attempting to recall visual symbols was helpful in designing this part of her therapy program. It allowed us to be efficient and effective in expanding her processing skills quite rapidly. Since there are a number of ways of teaching memory skills, it was important for us to understand how she was using her memory. We were then able to provide her with new strategies to change her ineffective, self-taught systems.

In order to develop strategies, we needed to understand the relationship between quantity of information which can be recalled and the complexity of the task being tackled. Both visual memory and language skills are essential for tasks which require symbol interpretation. The sequence appears to begin with seeing the stimulus, imaging or otherwise impressing the image on the memory, saying it with the inner voice and finally saying it aloud. This process appears to happen almost simultaneously for the skilled reader who is reading aloud. These are the steps that occur when the task is broken down or when a delay is inserted between stimulus and response.

To experience this, follow the steps below:

1. Look at the design at the end of these steps for five seconds.
2. Cover the design with your hand.
3. Wait thirty seconds.
4. Tell someone what the design looked like in enough detail that they could draw what you have seen.

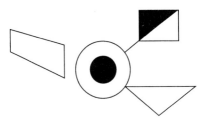

Most individuals find that they can study the design and image it, even when it is covered. If they were asked to write it down, they could do so quite easily (motor response). Instead they are asked to describe it in words. This means that they have to change it from a graphic symbol system to a linguistic symbol system. The verbal response is more difficult than a written response. This is also the processing pattern most frequently used by a beginning reader.

We can select a strategy for improving visual memory skills once we understand the strategies the individual has been using in attempts to remember. The main strategy for recalling visual information looks like the following:

See ⟶ Image ⟶ Respond (Write, speak, draw, perform)

This strategy with a verbal response is important for developing reading and spelling. Since the way we develop spelling skills is through seeing the words as we read, it is a natural way for increasing the spelling vocabulary. In the training programs reported in this section, the goal is to eventually teach the individual to use this technique. The most rapid reading and spelling growth occurs when this skill works on an automatic basis.

Other patterns can be used for processing, but tend to be useful for short-term rather than long-term memory. For *long-term storage*, the image or visualization step needs to be included in processing.

VISUAL MEMORY SEQUENCES

See ⟶ Verbalize ⟶ Respond

This strategy is observed with individuals who prefer to use their verbal skills. They tend to translate "seen" information immediately into words. This technique is often used best by individuals who have strengths in auditory recall. An alternative pattern for processing by individuals who use this pattern is *See➤Verbalize➤Image➤Respond*. It is the goal of programming to accomplish this transition.

See ⟶ Feel (Tactile/kinesthetic) ⟶ Respond

Individuals who learn through feeling, touching, and moving tend to try to use these strengths in memory for seen information. They will be observed writing with the finger on a table as they try to recall a sequence or sketching in the air. The most efficient pattern for them to develop will be learning to image with or without marking space. Their pattern would look like *See*➤*(Feel)*➤*Image*➤*Respond.* The two important aspects of the new pattern is the reduction in dependency upon tracing the image and the awareness of the visual image.

See ➔ Pictorial Association ➔ Respond

Some individuals like to make pictorial associations in order to recall information. They may image the object or scene and try to recall through this channel. It is reported as an interim step to recalling the symbol (letter) image. For instance, one individual reported that when she was asked to write the word "tree" she immediately imagined a tree. Then she had to replace that image with the word *"tree."* This pattern had an extra step which would look like: *See*➤*Picture Word*➤*Image*➤*Respond.* This pattern is inconvenient because of the additional step which decreases processing speed, but it may not create problems for learning. The key in this pattern is assisting the individual in making the word image. If the skills for pictorial imaging exist, they can be used as a basis or strategy for developing the image of the word.

See ➔ Language Association ➔ Respond

Language is also used for providing an association. The individual who uses language will usually interpret or relate what is being seen to an experience of memory. One client reported that when she saw the word kitten it reminded her of a Halloween story about a cat. When she saw the word kitten she frequently read it as *"cat."* The language association can take the individual off target as they think (inner dialogue) about it. Therefore, there may appear to be no relationship between the word which they are seeing and their response.

The most effective pattern strategy for individuals who work with language associations is to move them from the associative level to a verbalization of what they are seeing (description). Then work with the description until it can be visualized. It would look like *See➤Verbalize➤Image➤Respond.*

MEMORY LEARNING STRATEGIES

The human brain has many abilities which allow it to learn in new ways. Some learning strategies which are effective in increasing memory are included here to serve as samples. There are many more which can be created. It is essential to identify the pattern which works most efficiently for the individual. Then teach them to augment their system with a new strategy which allows them to control their memory. These strategies include the following:

IMAGERY
This strategy asks the individual to look at or study a visual image. With new learners, begin with simple line drawings of common objects and proceed to shapes, numerals, letters and finally words. Use a word with the digit span capability of the individual. For example, to teach a seven digit word "success" the following steps may be used:

Example with word success:
1. Look at the image of the word on this card until you can look up and still see the word on the wall in front of you.

Success

2. I will remove the card when you can see the word on the wall.

3. Point to each letter and spell the word from your image. (The accuracy of the visual recall can be immediately monitored with this activity. If there is an error in the image, repeat step one. If they continue to have difficulty, decrease the quantity (use fewer digits) or the complexity (go from
   letters to numbers or pictures).
4. I will ask you to work with your image of the word.
   a. Have them move the image to the wall on their right. (Typical questions: Tell me the second letter in the word, tell me the third letter from the right, move the image to the wall on your right.)
5. Put the word in front of you on the table and spell it as you trace the letters with your finger.
6. Write the word on a piece of paper.

This sequence is one of the more efficient for learning spelling words. The individual is using the same parts of the brain needed for reading and spelling. This activity utilizes all of the brain's resources (multi-sensory).

ASSOCIATION
In this technique, the individual uses known images to assist in retaining new information.

Example: Picture to Word Images
1. I would like you to tell me about your favorite car. Tell me what it looks like so I would recognize it if it were in the parking lot. Encourage them to use gestures and attribute (color, material, shape, size, etc.)
2. I would like for you to image a red balloon. Tell me what it looks like and show me how big it is. Now imagine the balloon with red stripes. On one of the stripes write the word red. (Dictate it if the student cannot spell the word.) Show me how you wrote the word **red** on the

balloon. Now let the balloon go and watch it go up into the sky until you cannot see it anymore. Tell me when it is so small that it is gone.

VERBALIZATIONS

When the language center appears to be stronger for the individual than the visual memory, teach them to use their language skills to "read" the visual image they are trying to recall. This is an especially useful technique when an individual has a word which they have learned incorrectly and they continue to repeat an error pattern. One student consistently spelled *girl* as *"gril."* After many errors, he developed the saying, *"a GI can be a girl."* From then on, he had no difficulty spelling the word.

The challenge with association techniques is that they are inefficient for general use. We cannot develop an entire reading vocabulary through associations. As a transition technique or for special circumstances, it is a good strategy and should be included as one of the choices for learning new words or recalling important information.

TACTILE/KINESTHETIC

Using motor memory to reinforce visual memory is very effective for many individuals. It appears that tracing over the image or writing it engages an important part of the brain in the learning process. Use the steps from the Imagery sequence. Reinforce by having the individual trace each letter with his index finger first on the card and then by tracing each letter on the image

IMPROVING MEMORY

These exercises will increase quantity of memory. If an individual can recall five items but their attempts to recall six are unsuccessful the following technique will assist. The doubling technique is successful and can be used for visual or auditory memory practice. Practice each step for several sessions before moving to the next step.

DOUBLING TECHNIQUE

The following steps have proven effective in order to increase the amount of information that individuals can recall:

1. Repeat after me 2-4-7-3-9.
2. Double the last two digits and say: Repeat after me 2-4-7-3-9-9.
3. When that step is successful, double the first two digits and say: Repeat after me 2-2-4-7-3-9.
4. When that step is mastered, double the middle digits and say: Repeat after me 2-4-4-7-3-9.
5. Now they are ready for six separate numerals.

MISSING PIECE

Individuals who experience memory inefficiencies with primacy memory errors are often helped by identifying the missing piece. In this strategy, they learn to focus on a the part of the information which has tended to confuse them before.

Steps for Improving Recall with Missing Piece Technique
1. Ask them to listen to a sequence of digits such as 24739. Then have them them tell the sequence again with some numerals missing–2 4 7. Have them recall what is missing and where they were in the original sequence.
2. Use a card with the numerals on it–2 4 7 8. Ask them to look at the card and then remove it. Have them tell you the last two numbers on the card.

   Training memory skills in isolation is not useful for improving reading and spelling skills. The memory training activities identified here are dynamic strategies which have utility for reading and spelling. While the initial tasks have the individual building on quantity up to eight digits, no improvement will be experienced in academic subjects until the strategies for using memory are used and practiced with spelling and reading words.

INTEGRATING PROCESSING SKILLS STRATEGIES

One of the most important aspects of the memory training and strategy program is teaching individuals to work with interference. If they can sit in a quiet room and repeat up to eight items correctly, that is only the very beginning. Since we are rarely required to remember something in quiet isolation, the training of tolerance for interference is an essential part of the memory development strategy. Interference strategies which we use include:

INTERFERENCE OPTIONS
Time Delays Individuals should be able to tolerate a ten to thirty second delay between seeing a stimulus and repeating or writing it.

VISUAL INTERFERENCE
Visual interference can be created by asking them to look at a stimulus and recall it while they place a piece in a puzzle (locate an item on a hidden picture, look at a number line, check a math problem for accuracy, etc..) and then repeat the stimulus item.

AUDITORY INTERFERENCE
Auditory interference requires them to look at a stimulus and recall it while they listen to someone repeat their address (spell a name, read a paragraph in a story, repeat a rhyme, etc.) and then repeat the stimulus item.

WRITING
Written interference asks them to look at a stimulus and retain it while they write some other information (write their name, phone number or address, copy a word, write a sentence, etc.) and then repeat the stimulus item.

MOVEMENT

Movement interference involves asking them to look at a stimulus and recall it while they stand up and walk around the chair (hop three times on one foot, go to the door tap the doorknob five times touch the floor return to the desk, or tap a rhythm, etc.) and then repeat the stimulus item.

VERBALIZATION

In this instance, individuals are asked to look at a stimulus and remember it while they talk about something else (spelling their name backwards, counting from one to ten, repeating a tongue twister, etc.) and then repeat the stimulus item.

The three phases of memory development include: increasing the quantity or number of items, developing a tolerance for interference and learning strategies for application to reading and spelling development. In preparing the brain for learning, both visual and auditory memory are major components. Auditory memory training parallels visual memory. The unique components are described in the following section. Techniques for improving memory and basic processing strategies may be adapted for visual or auditory training. The visual examples are not repeated but may be used as models.

AUDITORY MEMORY DEVELOPMENT

Individuals with auditory memory inefficiencies frequently report that they have difficulty in following directions, following a conversation, or listening to a lecture. They report that their spouses claim *"they never listen."* As children, they are frequently in trouble for forgetting to do what they are told. They often make errors in pronouncing sounds (articulation) or do not speak in full sentences (phrasal speech patterns). Individuals who experience the **Auditory Comprehension**

Confusion and those who experience **Attention Focus Confusion** frequently have auditory memory inefficiencies.

Patterns for developing auditory recall parallel those used for visual memory development. Obviously, the most skillful learners can shift between these processing patterns and adapt them to the type of situation or material they are using. The effective learner responds to visual as well as heard information with competency. He may prefer to learn in one mode or another, but is able to process in a variety of modes.

Since memory is not a subject which is taught in school, we have all had to develop our own techniques and resources for remembering as best we can. When we are working with individuals with inefficiencies in their processing we cannot assume that they know how they are processing or even how to do it effectively. This is the primary reason that we teach memory training as an essential part of preparing the brain for learning.

To experience auditory processing, ask someone to dictate the following exercise. Give them this page with the series of items and ask them to follow the steps below:

(Note: Be certain to pace the dictation of the items evenly at a two per second pacing and drop the voice at the end of the series.)

1. Say: " I am going to say a series of mixed numbers and letters. Please repeat them to me when I have finished each series.

    G 3 7
    F 9 S 2
    B 3 R T 5
    9 G W 3 1 H
    P 4 W S 6 8 2
    L Q 9 N 7 F 1 5

2. Provide a piece of paper and say " I am going to say a series of mixed numbers and letters. Please write them down when I have finished the series.

Remember to wait until I have finished.

M 2 J

S 4 3 L

G 5 9 W R

2 Y C 6 J G

R Q 4 P 3 1 8

T 7 E X 9 L M V

Discuss how you attempted to remember these series of digits with the person who assisted you. As you describe the pattern you used for memory, you will recognize you own learning strengths and the strategy you bring to a listening activity. You will notice how it may be different based on whether you could say the item or had to write it.

The most common and efficient pattern for auditory processing and verbal expression is one that stays within the verbal language system.

AUDITORY MEMORY SEQUENCES

Hear ⟶ ReVerbalize ⟶ Respond (Speak, Perform)

This pattern must be adapted for spelling tasks because they require the use of the visual symbol system. For efficient processing the pattern should include visual imagery.

Hear ⟶ ReVerbalize ⟶ Image ⟶ Respond (Write, Draw)

The skill for integrating what is heard and turning it into a visual image of words or pictures is essential for reading, writing, spelling and comprehension.

If auditory memory development appears to be weak, then the first level of training will need to be on the element of quantity or the number of items to be remembered. We do direct drill for training memory skills.

AUDITORY IMAGERY

In this strategy, the individual is being asked to construct a visual image through listening. Imagery training usually begins with descriptions of actual objects, places, events, etc. For instance an imagery at the concrete level could give the following:

1. The individuals are asked to imagine a cat. For this task they are asked to image with their eyes open, since we will eventually want them to develop this skill for spelling purposes.
2. Individuals are asked to describe the cat, tell where it is on their image screen and then move the image of the cat to the left side of their picture. Say, *"Tell me when you have placed the cat on the left of your picture."*
3. Ask them to imagine a tree on the right of their picture, then see the cat run across the space to the tree and run up the tree.
4. Ask them where the cat is now. Have them describe which side of the tree the cat climbed up and where it is located. What it is doing in the tree?

Once a visual imagery can be verbally guided, then the imagery techniques can be transferred to symbols.

1. Say: *"Listen to these letters and place them on your visual screen as you hear them: can."*
2. *"Are the letters still there?"*
   Affirmative response: *"Read them to me and point to where you see them at the same time."*
   Negative response: Reduce the number of items and repeat step one saying, *"Place a "c" on your screen. Is it still there? Point to it and trace it with your finger."*
3. Once the image has been placed on their screen, have them place their hands on both sides of the letters and

move the word down to a paper in front of them. *"Read the letters to me and point to where they are at the same time."*

4. Ask them to copy over the letters with a pencil or crayon and then ask them if they know what the word says. If so, ask them to read the word.

This activity in imagery can be done with nonsense letters, numerals or shapes. If an individual is especially sensitive about not reading, then it may be appropriate to use nonsense letter sequences until the memory is strengthened.

This is one of the most effective patterns for improving auditory memory with the intent of writing or reading. If the individual has difficulty with this pattern it may be appropriate to reinforce it with the TACTILE/KINESTHETIC pattern. To adapt this technique for auditory patterning, writing in the air or on an imaginary surface is used to reinforce learning.

ATTENTION FOCUS TRAINING

The purpose of attention focus training is to increase the length of time individuals can attend to a stimulus and to learn to screen out distracting stimuli. For our purposes the stimulus is reading, spelling, calculating, listening, writing, or thinking. It is important to understand several things about attention focus prior to beginning training efforts:

ATTENTION FACTORS
1. Attention skills will vary depending upon the object of the attention. Jill could give more attention to a film on raising horses than one on the Civil War. Scott could absorb every detail of a discussion about who should be the instructor for the class, but could not focus his

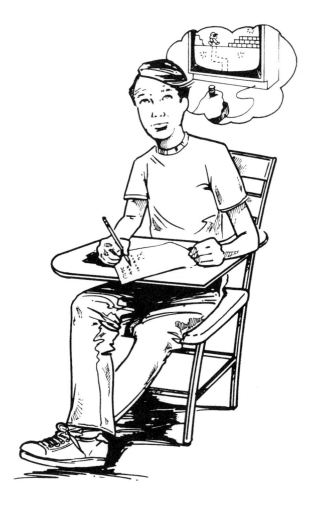

attention to listen to the instructor lecturing. Annie could draw and color a detailed picture depicting a field trip to the zoo, but couldn't complete her handwriting paper.

2. Individuals usually do not know when they have changed their attention focus. In other words, they do not consciously decide to stop paying attention. It just seems to happen to them. Therefore, they cannot control it and stay on task.

3. Attention is made up of multiple facets, including integrating what is seen, heard, felt and thought. If any of these processing systems are inefficient or significantly different than the others, the imbalance appears to distress attention skills. For instance, Carley can watch a dance step and recall every movement, but can keep her attention focused for less than a minute on listening. If a task involves a passive form of listening, her attention wanders.

4. The greatest challenge for attention is concentrating on passive or low interest stimuli. In other words, students can attend for long periods on items with high interest (computer games) but they have difficulty focusing their attention on materials and activities with a low stimulus value such as reading, writing or lectures. They become distracted by more interesting stimuli which can be internal (daydreaming) or external (someone walking by the room or activities outside the window).

5. Individuals with attention focus disruption often have the capacity to track multiple stimuli. Scott described sitting in class and tracking up to six interactions and activities at one time. He knew who was walking by in the hall, who had answered a phone in the room and what they were discussing, who the instructor was working with and what their problem appeared to be,

who got up to take a break and who joined them when they left the room. Everything that was going on in the room was noticed, except what was in the book in front of him.

We find that it is important for individuals who have attention focus challenges to discuss what they are experiencing. If it is a child, it is important for the parents and, if possible, the teacher to be involved in the discussion. Everyone needs to understand what they are experiencing, especially the individuals themselves. They need to understand that:

Important Observations About Attention:
1. Attention focus varies at different times and for different subjects.
2. Attention focus changes with such things as fatigue, nourishment, stress, and relaxation.
3. Attention focus is controllable with training.

ASSESSING ATTENTION SKILLS
In assessing attention is it appropriate to assess three factors.

1. How long can they sustain attention on a task with written materials?
2. Do they register when they divert their attention from the focus?
3. What are they focusing on (thinking about, looking at, etc.) when they divert their attention?

Adults can provide much more specific information than children regarding what they are experiencing. John realized that many of the arguments he was having at home were related to his difficulty in listening. When we explained to him what he was experiencing, he reported that he *"wished his wife could of heard that, cause then she'd understand."* At that point, he imagined her being there and listening to the conversation and reacting to it. His imagination was so vivid that he was not always aware when he was paying attention and when he had diverted his attention to an internal stimulus.

PREPARING FOR INTERVENTION

Most individuals we have worked with have been quite anxious to change their attention skills. Even those who were not convinced that they needed it became believers when they found that they could not maintain their attention on the balance beam for longer than thirty seconds. One ten year old boy told us that it was *"impossible for anybody to do go for more than ten seconds (his time) on the balance beam."* When we told him about students who can do it for seven minutes, he decided to take on the challenge.

Individuals are usually not aware that we can recognize when they stop paying attention. Since they do not identify when they move off-task themselves, they are surprised that someone else would know. We show them on the balance beam that when they start to think about something else that their eyes move. This is very easy to demonstrate by putting them in front of a full length mirror and asking them to maintain their eye contact with themselves as they walk forward and backward on the beam. If they still do not seem to be aware of the shift of attention, we will use a stop watch and click it when we see their attention shift.

TRAINING TECHNIQUES

We are using a combination of training techniques from three experts in the field. Each of these techniques emphasizes the integration of both sides of the brain. It is our goal to integrate balance with visual and auditory attention focus. Although each of the programs uses different terminology and has unique activities, each can accomplish the goal of preparing the brain for learning to attend.

These are all proprietary techniques and cannot be described in this text except as reference. We will explain how we are using them for attention training and for improving brain processing.

PERCEPTUAL MOTOR ATTENTION TRAINING

Formerly the Director of Perceptual Motor Therapy at the University of Houston College of Optometry and Professor of Developmental Psychology at Pacific States University, Dr. Frank Belgau now resides in Port Angeles, Washington. He has provided our staff with materials, equipment and an understanding of activities which improve basic brain function. For many years, we have utilized Dr. Belgau's training programs and equipment in our facility. He provides frequent workshops in the western states. Copies of his materials and a schedule of his workshops are available through the reference in the Materials and Program Appendix. Dr. Belgau wrote in his description of his program:

> *You can dramatically improve the brain functions that underpin vision, audition, motor coordination, reading, handwriting, and arithmetic by doing special brain integration activities. The activities involve a great deal of cross-model feedback. While you are doing the activities, your body is precisely centered and your level of balance is monitored and controlled. Centering is important because centering requires that the two brain hemispheres function in a synchronized manner temporally and spatially. Controlling balance levels is important because the level of integration in an activity is relative to the level of balance of that activity. The integration must become more precise and more refined for you to operate at higher levels of balance..."*

With perceptual motor training activities, individuals appear to be better able to sustain reading attention. We are very successful in having them transfer the attention focus skills to reading which also requires the integration of seeing, listening, recognizing rhythm and maintaining attention. In order to accomplish the transfer of the new skill, we discuss the similarities in brain function with the individuals and show them how to practice the attention tasks during reading.

Dr. Belgau provides an extensive series of exercises which can be adapted to this focus in his manual *A Perceptual Motor and Visual Perception Handbook of Developmental Activities for Schools, Clinics, Parents and PreSchool Programs.* For individuals with a dyslexic learning style, we have found the tracking activities suggested in this manual very helpful in increasing tracking skills and stabilizing the printed word.

We measure the length of time the individuals can maintain their attention focus on a target while maintaining dynamic (moving) balance. The steps which we have found successful include the following:

1. Have them walk on a low balance beam while watching an eye level X target on the wall. As they walk forward and backward on the beam, time the sustained focus on the target. When they look away from the target, the timing is stopped. (If they are unable to walk on the balance beam, an eight foot line of tape on the floor may be substituted for the beam and the same procedure followed.)

   They should be able to walk smoothly forward and backward on the beam while maintaining the focus point. Initially they may be able to maintain the focus point and balance for five to ten seconds. With several practice sessions, the time will lengthen significantly. Consistently chart the sustained time and involve the individual in the goal setting activity.

The stopwatch is used to provide feedback to the individuals regarding the amount of time their attention can be sustained. We position ourselves next to the focal point, so that we can see their eyes. If they avert their eyes from the target, other than in a blinking motion, then the stopwatch is stopped. This provides them with immediate feedback that they have changed their focus. Each time, inform them how long they sustained focus, *"You focused for thirty seconds."* It is important that it not be stated in a judgmental way. They are working on their own goal and will make the appropriate judgements internally.

2. As they maintain the focal point and continue moving on the beam, we talk about the feeling of *"being focused."* One of the major strategies which we are attempting to communicate is that maintaining a focus is beneficial. We want them to internalize the feeling of shutting out external stimuli and being focused on the visual target and the balance of their body in space.

   The dialogue which is used should provide positive suggestions such as: *You can feel that you are in control of your body and your attention. Nothing can bother you when you are keeping your attention. Whenever you choose, you can use your attention in this way. You can experience this feeling when you are working on a reading or writing task. You can accomplish all of your work when you are focused like this.*

It is essential that they understand that the purpose of this activity is to increase their attention skills and to transfer this skill to other tasks which require attention.

3. Once they can maintain a two minute focus/balance, then auditory processing is added to the task. They move forward and backward on the balance beam to a

simple four/four rhythm with eyes focused on the target. We use a metronome to provide a simple beat, since speed can be adjusted for comfort.

Many individuals find that they cannot maintain a rhythmic movement or walk to a beat. If necessary, we begin by having them walk across the floor to the beat. Some will find it helpful to clap the beat first and then move in a marching step. We always ask them to wait and feel the beat before they begin to move. The rhythm can be changed at appropriate transition points. Prepare for the changes, so that they can accomplish a smooth transition and continue maintaining their focal point. For instance the instructions may be, *"When you reach the end of the beam, you will wait for a new rhythm, continue to stay focused on your target, listen to the new rhythm until you are comfortable to move to it, then begin."*

Their goal is to sustain a comfortable movement to a beat with the attention focus on a target. With this integration of balance and auditory and visual skills and the integration suggestion, we usually begin seeing a transfer occurring in reading, also. The individual begins to report that they feel more organized and in control.

4. Once the individual is comfortable in working with these exercises, then a variety of other integrating tasks can be used. The variety is limited only by the imagination of the teacher. Two variations which we have found to be effective include:

a. As they move on the balance beam with focus on the target, give math problems for them to solve. Simple problems such as: 2 + 7, 9 +4, 6 x 7, etc. require listening and thinking as the individual maintains balance and attention. More sophisticated problems can be used as appropriate for each individual.

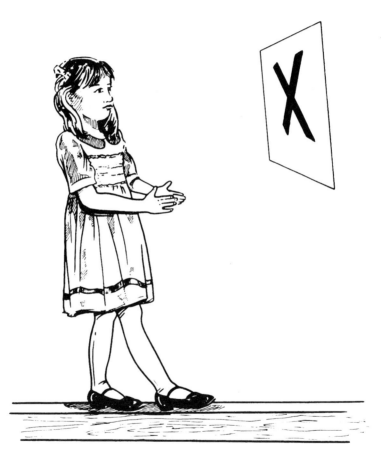

b. Ask them to image a word on the focal target and work with the word as they move on the balance beam. For instance, if the word is *"best,"* image the word on the target. Now as they move, dialogue about the word with questions such as, *"What is the first letter? What is the letter on the far left? What is the second letter? What is the sound of the letter on the end of the word? What do the last three letters say? What is the word?"*

When the individuals are integrating their attention, visualization, verbal processing and balance, they will be able to carry on this dialogue. Children, in particular, like to practice their spelling words through this type of a dynamic technique. They also find that they tend to remember them more effectively.

In order to achieve the desired improvement the teacher should assist them to focus attention on the task by saying *"just like when you are on the balance beam."* The teacher can time them for maintaining attention to the paper and pencil activity. In an effort to teach them to tune out distraction, the teacher may choose to introduce distracters into the activity and challenge them to stay focused.

Individuals who experience challenges in reading often have concurrent difficulty in integrating movements of body parts, including eye-hand coordination. A good example of the effectiveness of these exercises was an extremely intelligent twelve year old boy. Mark's intellectual scores exceeded 140 I.Q. on measured tests. He was very creative and loved to construct anything from forts and swings, to model planes. We always noted that masking tape and rulers would disappear with him and reappear as elaborately constructed jets or amusing sculptures.

When he walked down the hallway, it appeared as though his body parts were disconnected. Hands seemed to fling out, elbows moved in different directions and feet traveled independent of his body. As we began to do the attention exercises with him it became apparent why we had this image of him walking down the hall in pieces. He could not cross his midline without great effort. When he attempted to raise his left knee and tap it with his right hand (cross-crawl—which requires crossing his mid-line and coordinating both sides of his body), he could not be successful. He might, with great effort, tap it once, but when he tried to do the next move of right knee and left hand, his right knee would come up and his right hand would tap it. He consistently reverted to a homolateral (using one side of the body—left hand tapping left knee, right hand tapping right knee) pattern for this cross crawl movement. As he attempted to coordinate this movement, his posture would change. His knees would appear to sink and his back and shoulders would hunch forward. It appeared as though he were curling up before our eyes. He was aware that he was struggling, but was not aware of what was happening to his posture and control.

We placed a full length mirror in front of him so he could observe his posture. As soon as he saw himself, he began to take control of his posture. We had him do the cross crawl in front of the mirror in slow motion. We talked him through it to give him the rhythm of the synchronized movement. By the third practice session, he could perform the exercise comfortably. He would immediately control his posture with a verbal prompt to *"check your posture."*

He could walk the cross crawl on the balance beam by our fourth practice session and maintain his posture. The most unusual thing which happened was that he began to walk with control. He moved smoothly, appeared to know where all of his extremities were and could keep them under control.

He began to move smoothly in tracking the bean bag toss from one hand to another. He could track the moving ball and control its path while balancing on the variable balance platform. At the same time with a subtle prompt, he began to take control of his reading pacing and found that he did not lose his place as he was reading.

These activities are appropriate to use in any environment. They can be done with multiple students at one time. They can be done by a classroom aide or trained volunteer. These activities should be done on a daily basis until individuals master the control of balance, movement and integration of eye movement.

EDUCATIONAL KINESIOLOGY AND ACUPRESSURE

We began working with these concepts through information received from the Santa Cruz County Office of Education in 1985. Dr. Jeanne St. John, Project Pres. Director for the county office had brought acupressure techniques into the public schools with great success. We were very curious about the application for relaxation and improved attention skills.

This information was joined with the information from the Educational Kinesiology Foundation, established by Dr. Paul Dennison and Gail Dennison. They have developed a variety of materials and workshops which teach educators how to integrate movement and learning and benefit attention skills.

References for both of these resources are provided in the Materials and Programs Appendix.

The activities provided in the Dennison's book entitled *Brain Gym*, Teacher's Edition, are some of the most important resources. This resource provides a variety of exercises for stimulating different parts of the brain and increasing organizational skills. Both children and adults enjoy the movements and find that they can use them any time to improve their attention.

We have found that the activities integrate very effectively into the work we do in attention training on the balance beam. To enhance attention focus and expand the integration of movement, we frequently use the cross-crawl on the balance beam.

The Lazy Eight's movement, in which the client traces a large figure eight on its side (the infinity symbol), is found in both Dr. Belgau and Dr. Dennison's work. This is a good activity for integrating movements with both sides of the body and crossing the mid-line. The student tracks the hand as it forms the figure and improves eye tracking skills, as well.

Many individuals have experienced exciting results with the activities in Brain Gym. One nine year old student reported that he used the exercises each night to help himself relax and go to sleep. His parents were surprised to find him doing his exercises. He told them he felt better and felt like he was in control after he did them. He even showed them how to do the exercises he had learned.

DAVIS ORIENTATION COUNSELING PROGRAM

Our major focus on attention focus training began following our association with a unique, talented, dyslexic individual by the name of Ron Davis. Mr. Davis founded the Reading Research Council in Burlingame, California. As a dyslexic adult, Mr. Davis realized that he could control his dyslexic tendencies by controlling his perceptual disorientation. Since that time, he has worked with others with the same talents for pictorial conceptualization which he has experienced.

The intent of Orientation Counseling is to assist individuals in stabilizing their perceptions. Davis explains that the individuals frequently register what they think they have seen, as what was actually seen. Even when they look at the original perception again, they tend to review their perception rather than the actual one. This creates a false sensory perception.

Many individuals with a dyslexic learning style report seeing words *"running off the page"* or *"changing after I look at them."* This is related to the disorientation which Davis describes. Davis utilizes the "minds eye" to assist individuals in controlling their perceptions; thereby, stabilizing the printed word.

Once individuals can control the disorientation, Davis then teaches a word mastery technique to assist in correcting the faulty perceptions which have been collected while attempting to learn to read. The mastery technique impresses the correct word (or symbol) image through a unique technique. This includes developing the concept or understanding of the meaning of the symbol or word and making the symbols in a dimensional medium such as clay.

Davis believes that individuals with this talent in perception experience a low threshold for confusion. The threshold for confusion creates the tendency to disorient whenever conflicting perceptions are presented to the individual.

When an individual is feeling "oriented," the attention focus is well controlled. This was the observation which led to our intense emphasis on attention training for clients. Once we had experienced the difference in the ability of our adults who had experienced Orientation Counseling, we realized that the control of attention and perception were essential in a solution to the dyslexic challenge.

Scott, who shared his experiences with attention focus confusion, was very successful with the Davis Orientation Counseling techniques. When he first experienced the orientation counseling, he was a bit skeptical about it working for him. We did the orientation counseling with him and he was very polite. We felt that he could move his *"mind's eye"* quite effectively and that orienting him would be very successful. When we finished, he told us that he *"wasn't sure what it was all about, and he didn't think it would make a difference."* The next day he called on the phone with great excitement. He reported, "I tried what you told me yesterday and it seems to be working. I can screen out all the distractions around me and keep working." His greatest concern at that point was being able to keep his new skill. He was afraid that it would disappear.

Orientation training was very successful for Scott. He could work with greater concentration. When his children interrupted him, he no longer became angry and upset. He could tune out the sounds of their play. He no longer kept track of who was walking by in the hall or what his neighbors at other work stations were doing, except when he wanted to.

If Orientation Counseling is selected for improving attention training for an individual, it will require someone trained in the technique. Teachers and therapists may receive training in Orientation Counseling the Reading Research Council which is referenced in the Appendix. The techniques are also described in the recently released book *The Gift of Dyslexia* by Ronald Davis.

ATTENTION FOCUS REVIEW

In order to achieve the desired improvement in attention focus and integration of skills, individuals must understand the goals of the activity. The primary goal is to have them experience the feeling of being attentive and be able to return themselves to this level of concentration whenever they choose. The secondary goal is to have them recognize when they begin to disorient and choose to return to being focused.

Once they can control their attention, then the teacher will need to teach them when to use the control. As the student is reading or working math problems, the teacher can assist them in using their new skills by asking them to recognize their attention level. Suggestion statements such as, *"while you are working on this task you can feel yourself being very focused. You can stay on task without distractions."* are very effective.

For younger students, the teacher can help them recreate their attentive behavior by reminding them of the feeling of being organized on the beam. We ask them to recall how organized they feel when they are on the balance beam. Then we tell them:

> *Get in touch with how you feel when you are focused on the X on the wall. Pretend that there is an X on your work paper and concentrate on the paper as you work the problems. You will be able to tune out all distractions just like when you are on the balance beam. We will use a stopwatch and time your attention on the paper.*

With some students, we actually practice staying on task. We worked with a sixth grade student who continued to have serious difficulty in concentrating in a classroom. He was distracted and pulled off task by every movement or noise in the classroom. In an effort to teach him to tune out distractions, we chose to introduce distracters into the activity and challenge him to stay focused. We advised him that his job was to stay on task and continue reading aloud. We practiced reading aloud for one minute. Then we told him that this time we were going to create all kinds of distractions, but his job was to ignore them and stay on task.

He began to read aloud and we moved around behind him. We crushed papers, talked to the wall, moved boxes around and stacked interesting objects within his visual field. He continued to read and never skipped a word.

The next day we were passing his classroom where we could hear some talking and distractions occurring. He had turned in his desk to check it out. When he saw us, he smiled and gave a knowing look and turned around and continued to work. He stayed on task for the next fifteen minutes without becoming distracted or disoriented by the stimuli around him.

During our next session, we asked him why he had turned around in class and continued to work. He said that we had told him to get back on task and he did. We were surprised, since we had not even entered his classroom. This was pointed out to him and he seemed surprised to realize that he had taken his sighting of us as a signal to tune into his attentive behavior. He decided on a signal he could put on his paper, so that he could be reminded to stay on task when he wanted to finish his paper. He set a goal of working on his assignments for fifteen minutes and decided to use the clock on the wall to monitor his time.

One of the most important aspects of this interaction was the student's understanding that he was in control of his attention and his willingness to establish his own goals for improving his work habits. With students from ages ten through sixteen, one of the most important issues they work with is the issue of control. They frequently fight against the feeling that everyone is always telling them what to do.

One of the reasons that they feel "out of control" is because they are so totally at the mercy of external stimuli or internal distractions. They want to be "in charge," and they need to feel that they have gained power for themselves when they are able to attend to something. Once they experience this control, they realize that they are in charge of themselves and are willing to work at maintaining this feeling.

RHYTHM

Rhythm is one of the internal mechanisms which is often disturbed for many individuals with a dyslexic learning style. Moving to a beat or even maintaining a regular, rhythmic beat is difficult for them.

The relationship between rhythm and reading is subtle, yet essential. Reading has a distinct rhythm to it. Words are broken into syllables, words are aggregated to become phrases, voices rise and fall as they near the end of a sentence, words create increased paces as excitement builds in a selection. Poetry, rhyme and rap are all attractive and captivating because of the rhythm. All of these make reading enjoyable and interesting, but, more important, increase comprehension and understanding.

John, who shared his story in the Attention Focus chapter, had great difficulty with rhythm. He read in a monotone manner which tended to obliterate punctuation. His voice did not rise and fall in a rhythmic or melodic manner, and he did not feel the pause at the end of a phrase or a sentence. As a result, his comprehension suffered. He could just as easily have been reciting a list of words which had no relationship to one another. He learned to hear and repeat the rhythm in the spoken/read word first through repeating and moving to rhythms, and then by using the tapping strategy discussed in the next chapter. He felt that this played an important role in his progress.

Rhythm is taught first by integrating it in the attention activities. As individuals learn to walk on the balance beam and maintain attention, the rhythm activities are added to the sequence. Movement to a beat appears to develop an internal feeling of rhythm. The whole body must integrate and respond to the beat while maintaining focused attention.

Once the ability to respond to an external rhythm is achieved, individuals focus on maintaining an internal rhythm. A sample rhythm is tapped out, such as a simple 4/4 beat. Some find that it is easier to count out the sequence while others find it difficult to count and tap simultaneously.

A series of different rhythm patterns may be used. The variety is limited only by the creativity given to the instruction. The pattern should be repeated a minimum of ten times to be certain that it has been internalized and can be sustained.

Once individuals can tap out rhythms with several different patterns, they will also begin to be able to identify the syllables in a word. They can tap out the syllables as they hear them in the word and count the units. We vary the activity to include asking how many syllables are in a word, "How many beats (syllables) do you feel in the word baseball?" Sometimes we request the individual to provide a word with a certain number of syllables. *"Give me a word which has three beats (syllables)?"* or *"Which words have three beats? Breakfast, educate, literature, capital."*

When individuals have difficulty with rhythm in reading, we have them tap out each phrase by syllables. The rhythm for a sentence might look like this:

/ / / / / / / / /
If you go quickly, I will hurry, too.

These activities will assist in integrating the internal feeling of rhythm and the coordination of reading with the auditory system of the brain. Rhythm is an important processing skill and is helpful in developing reading competency.

SPATIAL ORGANIZATION

When they are asked to describe a dyslexic reading style, one of the first symptoms that most people think of are letter reversals. The confusion between letters like b/d or numerals like 5/2 or symbols like 9/p are frequently seen with beginning readers and individuals who experience a dyslexic learning style.

Ron Davis, of the Reading Research Council, describes the dyslexic individual as being talented in understanding the world in dimension. He finds that a dyslexic reader may look at a word from multiple perspectives when he attempts to read it. This act of seeing it from the left, from the right, and in dimension, may explain the feeling that the word changes or moves.

With the Orientation Counseling, Mr. Davis teaches the individual to stabilize the image or to see it from a consistent, centered point of reference. This is very effective for many individuals since it creates a reference point for looking at the words.

Similar results can be obtained with other attention focus training techniques. It is necessary to assist the individual who experiences this phenomenon in understanding what they are doing. This will allow them to recognize how it is happening and to take an active part in correction.

Young children often need to develop their spatial orientation skills so that they can experience the organization of space. The activities which benefit the early establishment of directional concepts are found in the work by Belgau, Frostig, Kephart, and many others. These three are referenced in the Materials and Program Appendix.

We begin programming with the identification of left/right, up/down and front/back spatial coordinates of the body. The most difficult is obviously the left/right identification. Individuals are guided through games and activities which have them identify left and right on their bodies. Gradually, we have them projecting it to describe spatial coordinates.

1. A suspended ball or tether ball can be used for developing beginning left/right awareness. We have the student tap the ball with their right hand, right shoulder, right knee, right hip, right foot, etc. They are developing a feeling of one side of the body before attempting to alternate or differentiate. If they experience confusion in maintaining lateral awareness of one side of the body, we provide them with a prompt-cue, such as a ribbon on the right wrist or ankle.

2. During the next session, we repeat the commands with the right side of the body. If they are comfortable in responding to the commands and are consistently choosing the right side, then we may introduce the *"other"* side. We have them tap the ball with *"your right hand, right foot, your other foot, your right hip, your other hip, etc."* We continue practicing for several sessions or as long as needed for them to make correct choices on an automatic level.

3. When they can perform #2 consistently, then we begin to substitute the term "left" for "other." They are asked to tap the ball with *"your right hand, right hip, right foot, your left foot, etc..."* Most individuals can make the transition quite easily, if they have first established #1 comfortably.

4. We provide the individual with a bar or stick which has a line or mark in the center. We tell them that they are going to use the right side of the stick to hit the suspended ball. We have them hold the stick with one hand on each side near the ends of the stick. (If necessary color cue the stick by painting the right side of the bar red and the left side green.) We then have them tap the ball with the part of the stick nearest the right hand. We can show them how the right side is the part from the middle line to the end on the right or how to keep a rhythmic tapping of the ball to keep it swinging smoothly. As they are

working with it, we refer to the "right" side frequently. *"You are hitting it with the right side very nicely. Keep the right side under control. The right side seems to be tapping the ball with a good rhythm."* The same progression as tasks #1-#3 are used in this activity.

5. Once individuals have a good understanding of left and right on the body and with items that are held by the body, then the concept should be taught as it extends into space. One simple exercise is to place them in the middle of a wall with their back to the wall. They should be focused across the middle of the room at an attention X on the far wall. They are asked to imagine a line that extends from the their noses to the X. We then ask the student to identify the right side. They are told that everything on the right side of the line is going to be on the right side.

We ask them to continue to keep their noses pointed to the X and to identify something on the right side. We are certain that their peripheral vision can pick up a variety of objects on the side. For instance, the instructor or a chair may be on the right side. We ask them to point with the right hand at the object he is identifying. Once this task is easy, then change the setting. We like to take the student outside and have them orient themselves from the mid-line by imagining a line from their nose to an object across a room, down the street, in a field, and then we have the student identify things on the right. We use the same strategy of *"on the right"* or *"on the other side"* before going to labeling the left side as identified in tasks #1-#3.

Adults with the dyslexic learning style will often complain about their skills in following directions or map reading. This same directional strategy can be applied to maps for adults who become confused about which way to turn when looking at a map. We teach them to orient themselves with the left and right in relation to the flat map surface. They may have to reestablish their mid-line several times as they make multiple turns to find a location on a map. As they chart their path, they can record the directions *"go to Maybury St. turn left, go to Main St. turn right, etc."*

Efficient processing skills provide a foundation for building reading skills. Individuals with inefficient memory skills or mis-perceptions of symbolic materials tend to continue to experience challenges in reading effectively. As basic processing skills become automatic, we advance to strategy training. The individual is ready to learn how to use their processing skills for learning and require the strategies for acquiring information.

Chapter Nine

Strategies That Work

A third grade girl spent hours copying her math problems each day during her math period. In fact it took her so long to transfer the math problems from the book to her paper, that she could barely began to solve the problems in class. Each night she had homework working the math problems from class. Her teacher and parents were very concerned because she spent so much time doing her daily work as well as the assigned homework each night. She was fatigued and rarely had time to play after school.

Her teacher observed that when she wrote down her problems, she copied one numeral at a time. She looked back at the book four times in order to write a problem with four numerals on her paper. In consulting the student's records, her teacher learned that she had experienced perceptual problems and early difficulty with visual memory tasks. While she now tested in the normal range on these tasks, she did not appear to be using her new skills.

During the spring of the year, she was referred for evaluation to the Learning Center for her arithmetic problems. It appeared that she had good knowledge of the number facts and understood how to use addition, subtraction, multiplication, and division processes with ease. Her only problem appeared to be her speed in working on her daily work.

Since her visual memory retained six items easily, it was determined that she needed to learn a strategy for using her visual memory for practical purposes. In just a few sessions she learned to look at the whole math problem, image the numbers and transfer the image to her paper. She enjoyed the challenge of trying to move longer sequences and found that she could easily transfer a three place plus three place problem with one look.

She agreed to use her new skill in math the next day and found that she could both write down the problems and work them very quickly. She was encouraged to write the problem and work it, so that she worked with the problem while she was most familiar with it. She reported that she could *"almost work it as she was writing it down!"*

To the delight of both her teacher and her parents, she completed her math paper in class. Her new strategies were only a beginning. She learned to use similar types of systems to assist in working on each of her subject areas. This reduced the homework load and provided her with much need time for play.

For many years, we have heard from educators that training of memory by recalling units or working on perception is ineffective. The primary reason that they find it to be ineffective is that they have worked with it in isolation. Typically, they set up a hypothesis such as *"Improving memory skills to six units of information will significantly improve reading scores."* If the hypothesis is successful, it is only because the subjects discovered that there was a connection between their new skill and their academics and made the application themselves.

Our math student provides us with an important example. She did not understand that because she had improved in her memory skills, she could use them for transferring information in math class. She had to be taught to use this new ability for a practical application. We find that once the individual's processing skills are beginning to improve, we must assume the responsibility of *teaching the strategies for application* to reading, spelling, writing, math, or whatever subjects have been frustrating due to processing inefficiencies.

Specific strategies which we teach to individuals with a

dyslexic learning style include the following: *Synchronization of Visual and Auditory Processing, Language Transformations, Logic application and Reasoning Skills, Time and Space Organization,* and *Study Skills.*

In working with individuals with dyslexic learning styles, we have found that these strategies are essential. There are undoubtedly additional strategies which may be taught. Techniques that were obvious and automatic for the traditional learner must be taught to the individual with a dyslexic learning style.

SYNCHRONIZATION OF VISUAL AND AUDITORY PROCESSING

One of the attributes which frequently accompanies Auditory Comprehension Confusion and Attention Focus Disruption is a dissynchronization in the transfer of visual and auditory processing. These readers tend to visually track the words more rapidly than they can be transferred for verbalization with the inner voice.

Many individuals report that they may be looking ahead at a word in the next sentence, while they are verbalizing a word in the middle of the prior sentence. The effect of this reading pattern is that words are substituted, misread, and omitted. The comprehension of information is severely distressed because of the errors.

John described an experience of tracking ahead as he was reading a sentence:

> *I was reading along and the sentence said, "They were nowhere to be seen, even though he kept feeling that they must be nearby." But what I read was, "They were now here to be seen, even though he kept feeling that they must be nearby."*
>
> *Instead of seeing "nowhere" I'd see "now here." And so that registered as the word to recognize, and it didn't make any sense in the sentence.*

He was visually looking far ahead of where he was verbalizing (comprehending) and had lost the correct registry of the word. This lack of synchronization in seeing and saying the words created significant confusion. The problem with this type of reading problem is that there are many times when the errors are made, but the reader misses it because the it still made sense in the sentence. When individuals attempt to read specific information, such as directions, instructions, and multiple choice or true false test questions, these types of errors cause frustration and confusion.

There are three strategies we use in order to improve comprehension in reading: Neurological Impress Reading, Tapping and Phrasing.

NEUROLOGICAL IMPRESS READING

R.G. Heckelman reported on the neurological impress method in an article in Academic Therapy Quarterly in 1966 (pages 235-239). We have been using it since 1968 and have consistently found it to be an effective strategy in improving reading. It is especially useful in establishing a synchronization between what is being seen and vocalized.

In this strategy, the individual and instructor read the same material aloud together. Initially, the instructor moves his finger under the words in a smooth manner and at the pace of the reading. Eventually the individual may take over the tracking responsibility. Heckelman cautions the instructor to pay attention to the ends of the line on a page to assure that the hand moves quickly back to the next line without interrupting the flow of reading.

This choral or joint reading activity should take fifteen minutes a day for enough days to provide eight to twelve hours of practice. The strategy can be taught to parents, teacher assistants, or older students selected by the individual, so that training can be maintained between therapy sessions.

We have always found this to be a useful strategy because

the individual is seeing the word, hearing it, and saying it all at the same time. Since the instructor is reading the words with the individual, the pressure for trying to figure out the word is removed and attack errors are eliminated. Therefore, they are rehearsing the correct reading of each word. Individual comprehension is also enhanced, because the words are heard with appropriate rhythm and expression

The instructor must resist the urge to give word attack instructions or ask them to figure out a word as they are reading. If they slow down on a word the instructor should take the lead and say the word. If they appear to be comfortable with the vocabulary, the instructor can echo or lag slightly behind their reading.

The instructor refrains from quizzing about what was read, but does permit them to volunteer any information they wish about the reading. The instructor will want to comment positively on the fluency with which the client is reading.

John reported that it took several sessions of fifteen-minute practice sessions before he began to feel comfortable with the choral reading strategy. Then it was very helpful to him.

> *I know when we started to read in sync, it was very uncomfortable because I couldn't really catch on to the pace. I'd just say the words in almost a monotone expression to get the pace going.*
>
> *Once I got to hearing the grouping of the words and the expression flowed into them, it really gave good meaning. When I read alone, my monotone was boring. I could hear myself speaking out loud, reading out loud, and I'd think about it and then I'd pull myself off track. I started thinking too hard; this doesn't sound right, it doesn't flow well.*
>
> *Now I'm not concerned about the flow of it. I can just read it for the words. It's just like we are talking and I read to the end of a breath and that's it. Because breathing has an aspect of verbalizing, it sounds very natural.*

This technique is especially useful when used in conjunction with the tapping technique which we developed to assist individuals in monitoring their pacing and tracking for reading.

TAPPING TECHNIQUE

Most readers with a dyslexic learning style are unaware of punctuation. It does not appear to have any importance in the sentence except for, as one individual reported, *"taking up space."*

In reality, punctuation gives important information in a sentence. It separates ideas, tells us when we are reading a question, indicates emotion, advises us when we are going to see a listing of words, etc. The punctuation guides the rhythm of the sentence and tells us when to drop our voices as we conclude a thought.

The tapping strategy makes the individual aware of punctuation and its importance in written communication. It requires that the individual pace in synchrony both visually and verbally.

When individuals are reading, they are asked to tap twice for punctuation marks including: commas, periods, question marks, exclamation marks, colons, and semicolons. We request that each punctuation mark be indicated by a double tap. This provides a comfortable rhythm to the reading.

Since the client must wait until they have reached the end of the phrase or sentence before tapping, it prevents them from tracking ahead to the next sentence. This synchronizes the eyes and voice and appears to dispel the energy which sometimes is created when just trying to "slow down."

The tapping also appears to help in chunking information for retention and enhances recall. Most of the adults who learn to use this strategy to develop pacing skills report an immediate improvement in their comprehension. They find that they are less likely to become distracted as they are reading. The active involvement of the motor task seems to keep them focused on the sentence.

Scott shared his feelings about gaining rhythm in his reading through the tapping technique:

I wished that I had learned this a long time ago, maybe coming to the realization about tapping the relationship of speed of reading. I know that everybody thinks that speed is better, you know, the faster the better type of thing. But you know, getting something out of what you read is a lot better.

When I grew up it was at a time, especially in high school, when everyone was talking about speed reading. There were always ads on the radio. I wanted to go through one of those classes because I knew how bad of a reader I was and I figured, hey, I'll learn to read so fast I won't have to worry about school work or any books. I'll just speed read the whole book and boom, I'll be set.

It probably wouldn't have done me any good as I think of it these days. I was probably reading so fast with my eyes anyway, it wouldn't have made any difference. But realizing that I can pace myself and realizing tapping and being on point, and all these little tools, have really, you know, helped me a lot. You know, I would take this tool, like the tapping, and go home and use it and put that tapping to work, magically, without even thinking about it. It was just natural.

The most interesting aspect of the tapping technique is that it appears to become an internal regulator after a while. The individuals do not need to tap in order to regulate the pacing of the reading and create the synchronized feeling. However, if they feel stressed with especially difficult or complex materials, they find that if they use their tapping strategy they can quickly return to their comfort level of reading with increased comprehension.

As they improve in reading and work with their synchronization techniques, then they need to become familiar with the natural phrasing which occurs in speech and is recorded in written material.

PHRASING

The written word tends to imitate the spoken word. Interestingly enough, the spoken word is controlled by our breath control. Our phrasing tends to be in relatively short bursts which can be uttered prior to running out of air. An effective speaker tends to group his or her words in chunks which, when completed, communicate the message.

In order to hear the spoken word as we read we must group the words into meaningful phrases. For instance, the phrasing below does not communicate the message which was intended.

> **Really this**
> **is very**
> **important and I for**
> **one am**
> **very concerned.**

The reader who has spent years in attempting to decode words and/or struggling with understanding the printed word has not seen the connection between speaking and writing. This is readily apparent in the student's attempts to write stories. The stories tend to merge one sentence or thought into another. Some stories have no punctuation, but each thought is connected with *"and."* This is a good indication of how they are processing written language.

In order to teach the phrasing strategy, we choose a well written page at the appropriate reading level. Then we mark on the page with a / after each of the phrases. We demonstrate reading the sentence or paragraph out loud with pauses at the / marks. The individual then reads the selection imitating the instructor. The text might look like this:

> **Really! / This is very important. / And I / for one,**
> **/ am very concerned. /**

Once individuals understand the phrasing which makes reading understandable and improves communication, they are then instructed in marking the phrasing. In order to assist in this activity, we may read the sentence out loud, exaggerating the phrasing for them. There are often different ways of dividing a sentence and they are encouraged to mark it as they hear it. This assists in building confidence and independence in skills.

Like the neurological impress reading and the tapping strategies, the phrasing is designed to develop automatic skills. It should not become an end in itself. We are responsible for assisting the individuals in assimilating the strategy and experiencing comfort with reading at which point it is no longer needed. This is a strategy for establishing competency in reading.

LANGUAGE TRANSFORMATIONS

To assist some individuals in succeeding in reading, it is essential to teach the transformations in the English language When most people read, they find that they can anticipate the next word. For instance if a sentence is being read and a word is blurred or missing, we can provide an effective guess to fill in the space.

The plume tailed _____ chased the mouse around the kitchen.

Be careful when you _____ the street at the busy corner.

We can easily fill in *"cat"* or some other creature from the information in the first sentence because we know that it will be some type of animal from the cues. We also know that it will be a noun and not a verb that we will be filling in. As a result, we can predict or anticipate the next word.

In the second sentence, we will be filling in an action word.

We may not be certain if the word is *"cross."* We may have filled in with *"walk"* or with *"clean"* or another word. When we are not certain, we will have to rely on secondary clues. Since in reading we are provided those, even if we do not automatically know what the word is, we will be able to guess accurately as soon as the first letter or first two letters of the word is seen.

Individuals who experience different patterns of speech or who have challenges in the verbal and grammatical construction of spoken speech will not readily be able to anticipate standard English construction. If the verbalization for describing a trip to a store sounds like, *"We is gone to store."* Then it may be difficult for them with their reading difficulties, to automatically guess or anticipate the words for the sentence, *"We are going to the store."*

Inefficient language skills are frequently seen with individuals with Auditory Comprehension Confusion. The expression difficulties are often challenging to discern because of the minimal language usage the teacher or therapist may hear. Some of the clues we see quite frequently are:

Phrasal Speech
Numerous repetitions of short phrases are evident in listening to the individual. A repetitive pattern such as: *"You got it"* or *"Yeah"* may be heard. When a question is asked or a description requested, then it is given in short phrases.

> **Q: "Where were you this afternoon?"**
> **A: "The store." (Instead of "I was shopping at the super market.")**
> **Q: "What did you buy?"**
> **A: "You know, just stuff."**

Written Language
A writing sample reveals the internal language that they experience. Frequently there are run-on sentences and omis-

sions of punctuation. The writing may communicate what happened, but the reader finds himself filling in or guessing at the sequence of events. The writing often requires the reader to guess the pronoun references.

> *Went fishing Sunday at a lake in the rain and the fish didn't bite so we went back and the cabin didn't have any wood so we chopped it up and forgot to open the chimney block and smoked it out.*

Grammatical Errors

Listening to the individuals reveals noun/verb agreement and other errors. These are more frequently heard with younger children, but can remain into adulthood. More often, as the individual gets older, certain acceptable phrases are repeated and the language becomes more limited in its variety.

These errors are readily apparent during testing, listening and observing of the individual with a dyslexic learning style. If such challenges are present, then it is important to include programming to assist in the grammatical transformations.

We utilize the program called "Ready, Set, Go For Language Competency" which begins with the simple practice of noun verb statements, then progresses to asking a question and answering with affirmative and negative statements. Other beginning level transformations are also covered. There is a great deal of practice and spontaneous speech required in the activities after the individual has learned the correct pattern. We then integrate the concepts into both reading and writing in order to complete the speaking/reading/writing circle.

Specific resources and materials that are useful in developing client skills, are identified in the Materials and Programs Appendix.

Since the purpose of strategy training is for ultimate use in the academic or living activities, the transitions from being able to speak correctly to reading are essential. When the individuals can identify the correct transformations in verbal language, then they need to begin to identify those same transformations in the material they read. It is appropriate to have them look through a page of text and mark the patterns they have just learned. For instance if they have just studied the negative response, *"No, I do not see a cat."* Then we choose or create some material that has the pattern in it and have them find it.

Another strategy for assisting in recognizing the value of anticipating the common transitions in language is to choose some "cloze" tasks. These are activities in which the individuals attempt to fill in a word from the context clues. The materials can be constructed to work with a specific pattern or general materials can be used. For instance in the example above, a cloze activity could look like:

No, I do _____ see a cat.
No, I ___ not see a dog.
No, ___ do not see a bird.

These types of activities can be varied with the language, age, interests and sophistication level of the individual. The importance of the language training as a strategy is relating it to the reading and writing activities that the individual is required to perform.

USING LOGIC–VERBAL AND VISUAL

We find it important to teach reasoning skills. Individuals who have found it necessary to utilize one learning channel more than another have often developed unique ways of reasoning. Good skills in reasoning require balance in processing through both visual and auditory channels. We begin with the reasoning activities which work with attribute materials. These materials begin with identifying three different categories: shape, size and color. Individuals sort these into a variety of categories to show the differences.

Once they can reason using concrete objects and verbally explain what they are doing, then they are ready to move into both verbal and visual logic materials. Midwest Publications publishes the most appropriate collection of these materials. Some of the most effective include:

Verbal Reasoning Skills
Visual Thinking skills
Analogies A, B, C, D
Mind Benders Series A
Verbal Sequences
Figure Relations

These materials teach problem solving. They assist in increasing vocabulary and categorization abilities. They teach visual manipulation of objects and analysis, and improve reasoning ability.

Reasoning skills are necessary in learning for comprehension, composition and solving arithmetic problems. As we have discussed with all strategies, it is important to point out the skill to the individual and demonstrate to them how the new skill can be used for academic purposes. For instance if the individual can solve a Mind Bender reasoning problem, then present them with a word problem in math and ask them how they would solve this problem. The important part of this is applying the strategy for a practical use.

ORGANIZATION OF TIME AND SPACE

The time and/or space confusion which is often present with the dyslexic learning style is one of the most frustrating symptoms. Adults and children both experience the chaos of living in a disorganized environment. They may be further stressed by a faulty internal time clock which often "fakes them out" when they try to gauge or estimate the passing of time.

TIME CONCEPTS

Children are especially confused with this concept. It is irritating to both teachers and parents. Individuals confuse the concepts of time (minutes, hours, days, weeks, months, seasons and years). Frequently they cannot recite the days of the week or months of the year. They are unable to anticipate when something will be happening. Since they cannot track time, they do not know when to hurry or when they can relax.

Adults appear to settle in to their estimate of time and seem to either be "unconcerned" with time or constantly "pressured." They experience great difficulty with the concepts of deadlines in work. They work at a frantic, frenzied pace or appear to be unaware that a deadline is approaching. They receive numerous complaints about being late for appointments or being "ready" on time. Spouses often report that they adapt to their mate's time confusion by telling them they have to be ready earlier. This way, they have enough time to "be late and still be on time."

Time must be experienced both conceptually and physically. The concepts of time are appropriately taught by constructing a calendar around a circle. They can then use this to find the quadrants which represent the seasons and add pictorial references to show the seasons. They can then add holidays and locate important family events like vacations and birthdays.

A twenty-six year old office worker experienced great confusion with deadlines and schedules in her work. In order to guide her in developing time concepts, we talked about the four seasons and how they were a quarter of a year. She then made a large circle out of the clay and divided it into four quarters. She selected something that she associated with each of the seasons: a flower for spring, a leaf for fall, a snowman for winter and a sun for summer and placed them sequentially in the four quarters. She chose to make her labels (fall, winter, spring, summer) in clay and then made a large label (seasons) for the whole scene.

When she had completed the task, she shared an experience she was anticipating which would be coming in the next season. As she was talking about it, she looked at her clay model and began to laugh in a delighted manner. She said, "You know, this is the first time that I could see how long I would have to wait for my trip in the spring. It doesn't seem so far off now that I can see it."

In addition to the conceptual understanding of time, we work with timers and stopwatches. We teach skills in estimating and being able to anticipate time. The units which we work with begin with seconds and minutes and extend to hours. We talk about how long a minute is and watch it on a watch or clock with a second sweep hand. We do activities in which the individuals learn to estimate the amount of time passing (in units from ten seconds to two minutes).

We talk about the pacing of the seconds and work in counting them off so we can anticipate or guess how much time has passed. A simple pacing technique for monitoring seconds is counting 1001, 1002, etc. while watching the clock. This pacing task also builds in a body rhythm, which benefits the sensitivity to rhythmic movement.

Once individuals can pace-count, then we remove the stopwatch from their view and have them tell us how much time has passed. *"Count the seconds until I tell you to stop, and we will see if you are in synchrony with the stopwatch."* We can also ask them to tell us when ten seconds have passed, *"Tell me when you think ten seconds have passed, and I will stop the watch and we can compare your time."*

The activities on the balance beam are integrated with this learning activity. We have them walk the beam at a pace of one step per second or one step every two seconds. We encourage them to count out the pacing and maintain their consistency in attention focus simultaneously.

Since this is an important strategy, it must be integrated

into useful tasks for academic and living environments. Students frequently have challenges in estimating how much time a homework task will take. They lose their attention focus and time passes while they are "out" and then they do not complete their tasks. They have difficulty in planning for when to do their homework or projecting deadlines, including daily ones.

With individuals of school age, it is essential to work with them on academic tasks as they maintain a conscious awareness of time. For instance: 1) Place a timer in front of the students and ask them to read for one minute or 2) Give the student a stop watch and ask them to time how long it takes to read one page.

These types of activities can be very effective in helping the student become aware of the passing of time. We frequently encourage parents to purchase a kitchen timer and set it for a ten minute period for their child to work on a homework task. When the timer buzzes, the child is asked to set it for a ten or fifteen minute break period to reward themselves for staying with the task. Several benefits are found with this activity. The child will usually be willing to work for the set period of time. The ticking of the clock keeps their attention focused. Finally, the child begins to get a sense of how much time ten minutes feels like.

Students also need to develop their own time lines. We ask students to prepare a weekly timeline. The time line has school and social activities on it. Each day is divided into hour blocks and a weekly scheduled is planned. One of the feelings that the student with time confusion experiences is that *"all I do is work."* It is important for the student to see the open time as well as the work time blocked on the schedule. They can learn to anticipate rewarding experiences such as free time or special activities, as well as balance their school assignments. Once they have planned their week out graphically, then it should be discussed with them. They can learn to "see" their week without having their schedule immediately in front of them and can describe the activities for the next day to their instructor. This integration of mapping the week, anticipating it (verbally and visually), and experiencing it is essential for teaching time.

Adults can use these same types of aides to improve their concepts of time. They frequently have greater ingrained habits for measuring time passage than younger clients; therefore, they will need to specifically identify the benefits of improved time concept understanding. Once they have worked on activities such as were described above for a six week period, they will find that their habits have changed and they are integrating their new skills without conscious effort.

SPACE ORGANIZATION

Individuals with the dyslexic learning style may find that they are at the extremes on the continuum for organizing their environment and their work. Some individuals are compulsively neat and organized. Those who live with them, parents, siblings, roommates or spouses, know that it is unwise to move things or to invade their private space. These individuals have found that they can maintain their structure by keeping it exactly the same.

One parent shared an experience they had when their child was just three years old. The mother, a single parent, enjoyed bringing home a miniature toy horse as a special treat for her son. The boy loved the horses and kept them on a shelf on display in the living room. Whenever his cousins came over to play, they took the horses out and after playing with them, left them strewn all over the room. Each time this occurred, the boy would painstakingly take each of the horses and place them back on the shelf.

One evening the cousins left very late and the boy was so tired she suggested that he put them away in the morning. He wanted to do it then, but finally was persuaded to go to bed. That evening the mother cleaned up and put the horses carefully on the shelf.

The next morning the son came into the room and looked in horror at the horses. He started yelling, "How could you do this? You put them all in the wrong places. Don't you know the gray one goes here and the black one has to be next to brown one. You messed everything up."

The mother shared her surprise over his reaction to her efforts, but in retrospect was even more shocked over what it told her. At age three, he had a very specific organizational plan which he could replicate. He knew exactly where more than thirty items belonged. His visual planning and organization were exceptional. This continued to be an obvious talent even now that he was in high school.

In contrast, many individuals with the dyslexic learning style find that they operate on an "out of sight, out of mind" organizational style. They are interested in and work with the materials which are in front of them, but they have no recall of what other materials they need or how they could be helpful to them.

Students recall getting a study guide, but have no idea where it might be. They are certain that they finished the assignment and must have turned it in (*"The teacher must have lost it."*), until they find it at the bottom of their locker. Teachers and parents alike despair when students forget to take home the text for their homework and can't recall any book report being assigned. While some of these issues are related to the issue of time, most are related to organizational skills.

We find minimal success in intervening in this area of development until the student decides that it is important. A teacher or parent feeling that it is important will not necessarily motivate the student. It is helpful to recognize and to identify the reinforcers which the student assigns to not doing the homework or assignments. Frequent themes we hear are issues of control and helplessness. It sounds something like, *"Everybody is always telling me what to do and I am sick of it. It's not their homework. Everybody yells at me cause I don't do my assignments. So it doesn't matter anymore if I do it or not, I'm always wrong. I can't be successful."*

Once the issue is identified, some specific counseling discussions may assist the student in seeing what they are doing. We talk with them about "power." They need to understand that they are in charge of their own choices. Whichever decision they make, to bring my book home or forget to bring my book home, is their decision. They really are in control.

One of our most difficult tasks is convincing a parent who is hooked on rescuing their child that the child is making conscious choices. Students who have parents that run around monitoring their homework and pressuring teachers to provide elaborate checklists and extra copies of assignments, have no need to be responsible for themselves. They are being taught that others will take care of them and do it for them if they refuse to be responsible or act helpless.

Many of the students feel that they will be unsuccessful anyway; therefore, they are helpless in making a change. Students who believe that they are helpless and not in control count on "luck" to get them through. Luck may take the form of the teacher forgetting to ask for the assignment, asking easy questions on the test, forgiving the student and accepting an "excuse" that usually accompanies not completing an assignment.

Once they decide to substitute the power/control model for the helpless/luck model, they are ready for goal setting. Once the student has decided that there are benefits to him in improving organizational skills, then the success rate is quite high when the parent supports the goal of independent, responsible behavior.

Organizational skills include developing a system for maintaining ones papers. There are a variety of ingenious folder devices which may be chosen by the student. Others may wish to design their own unique system. It is essential that they make these decisions, so they retain ownership.

These organizational systems are equally useful for adults as well as students. Adults often enjoy purchasing elaborate organizational date books. Others like to set up systems where they record their priorities on a "whiteboard" or planner sheet. Whatever they enjoy, they will use.

To reinforce organization the instructor may ask the student to visually locate where each of her textbooks are at present. When the student can image her locker, desk, room, etc. to locate materials, then it is apparent that she has an active and practical organizational system operating.

One additional technique has been very effective for students who have trouble getting organized to do their homework. When the student comes home from school, he sets up his homework as though he were going to do it then. He opens the book, heads the paper, has the pencil ready. He then leaves it as is and goes ahead with whatever activity is scheduled for after school: game practice, free time, music lessons, etc. When it is time for the student to do the homework, then everything is preset and it is much easier to move into a working mode.

Several executives we work with have chosen to use this technique in preparing themselves for writing reports, answering letters, etc. It eliminates the need to organize when one is ready to work and makes preparing to get started a pleasant, non-stressful experience.

STUDY SKILLS

It is important to teach study skills to students (elementary through college) with the dyslexic learning style. The study skills which are beneficial include: composition, note taking, and test taking strategies. A variety of programs have been referenced in the Materials and Programs Appendix.

It is especially helpful if teachers who have students with unique learning styles in their classrooms, investigate different ways of helping students gain information. We cannot assume that everyone comes to school with the skills to take notes or to write a composition.

If a teacher will lecture and outline major points on the chalkboard simultaneously, they will be amazed at the improvement in participation and understanding all students will demonstrate. Skilled teachers often demonstrate some type of "mind mapping" skills as they are lecturing in order to engage student interaction. Once the students understand how to graphically and visually chart the information, they can record the information for themselves and they experience active involvement in learning.

When we begin to work with an individual, we start by explaining how the brain works in receiving information. If we "told" them about it, the majority of our population would "vague out" early into the explanation. Instead, we draw the information and explain it as we draw. For example: an explanation on reading will usually begin with a drawing of the brain inside a head that is looking at the words in a book. As we talk about the visual center of the brain, we point to it and draw it. By the time we have finished the discussion with the diagram, the individual can usually repeat it.

One of the first activities we do with our intensive clients is to provide them with this explanation and the diagram. At their first staffing, we ask them to explain it to their parents or the clinic staff. Along with their presentation of their goals, this is an important part of their presentation. It demonstrates that they are aware of what they want to accomplish, that they are focused, and that they are in control.

Study skills and writing techniques must be taught to individuals with dyslexic learning styles. It cannot be assumed that because a student is in high school or because an individual holds a responsible job that they have these skills. Most of them have found alternative ways to "get by" which are inefficient and marginally effective.

Students can learn to write basic essays by understanding

simple charting techniques. Teachers need to be skilled in showing several different methods for constructing an essay. For instance, the Venn diagram format is an excellent way of developing a compare and contrast essay. If a student has to compare two characters in a book for a book report, the Venn diagram will assist them.

John was tall and regal in his carriage. He appeared to look down his long nose at the servants and the village people. They were frightened of his power although he never appeared to use it. Possibly, it was because he rarely spoke except within the family. That seemed to be why there were all surprised when he donated much of his wealth, upon his death, to establish a home for abandoned children.

His brother, Richard, bore a strong family resemblance to his sibling. It was not that he did not have the same aquiline features, it was the way in which he carried himself. It was possibly the smile which spread across his face and lit the twinkle in his eyes. He was consistently surrounded by children who enjoyed his funny tales and creative wit.

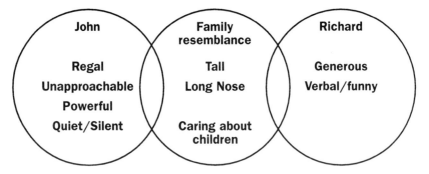

The information gained in this manner provides the student with the contrasts between the two characters. It gives them the characteristics which were the same. With simple assistance in formatting, they will have a frame with which to approach any type of essay which requires discussion of similarities and differences.

168

There are a variety of these types of organizational formats which will assist students in expressing themselves effectively in both written and verbal presentations. Once they know some of these logical systems, they can apply them to papers, essay questions and speeches.

These are a variety of strategies which improve learning. For individuals with dyslexic learning styles, these strategies must be taught and rehearsed. The application of these skills may not be automatically generalized to other learning experiences; therefore, they should be taught. It seems that strategies which most people learn as they mature, must be taught to students with dyslexic learning styles. We can not assume that because they can now remember more effectively, pay attention for longer periods and understand their spatial environment that they will now be able to read, write and perform academically. It is essential that they be taught the strategies for gaining information and using it. This requires the creative observation and ingenuity of the instructor. Each individual will be different and have different needs or possibly the same needs at different levels. In our last chapter on remediation, we will review some of the materials or programs which are effective in providing a system for reading and learning for the individual with a dyslexic learning style.

Chapter Ten

Reading Strategies
That Work

There are several reading systems with similar structures that work effectively for individuals with a dyslexic learning style. Some are more effective with specific learning styles than others. A variety of techniques which are commonly used in remedial reading programs are counterproductive to learning for these individuals. Among these are techniques that emphasize a sight/word approach, which relies on whole word memory skills. Literature programs which do not have concurrent phonetic instruction and programs that do not include the use of multiple senses are not effective.

Annie experienced a reading program which relied on whole word recall with reinforcement from flash cards. The failure she experienced with this technique caused her to experience serious stress and frustration. Her mother shares their experience with a sight/word program.

She has seen the same word on the flash card at least five hundred times and she still doesn't recognize it. It is as though she had never seen it before. We sit down every evening after dinner and go over the words just like her teacher suggested. Sometimes she recognizes them and other times it is just frustrating.

Sometimes we both end up crying. Sometimes it's just Annie. More often it's me. I just feel so bad for her. I know how important it will be to her to be able to read. I know that she knows, too. She loves books.

We hear parents and clients saying the same thing over and

over. The least effective technique for teaching an individual with a dyslexic learning style is flash cards.

It has always seemed common sense to us that if a person has not been able to learn with a specific technique, that fact should be accepted. A different technique or program should be used. We have to find a way that they can learn. A variety of reading systems have the teacher recycling the program over and over. We consistently ask, *"If it didn't work the first time, why are you using the same system again."*

The answer we are given is *"because they need lots of repetition."* This is definitely a myth for the dyslexic learning style. The reason that the technique is not working for them is because it creates confusion for the individual. It is not being integrated in the various areas of the brain which are responsible for retention of written words. Continually repeating something which does not work only creates frustration and failure.

The most important part of our work with individuals who have dyslexic learning systems is the selection of a successful system for reading. Several systems work effectively. We use the one which most appropriately matches the learning style of the individual. If we find that it is not quickly successful, we will augment the system with elements from others until we achieve success.

READING SYSTEMS

These are systems which we have found to be successful for reading development for individuals with different learning styles.

VISUAL SYMBOL CONFUSION
    Easing Into Reading
    The Auditory Phonics Program (TAPP)

Auditory Discrimination in Depth
Glass Perceptual Conditioning Program
Orton Gillingham Approach (Slingerland)

AUDITORY COMPREHENSION CONFUSION
Neurological Impress Reading
Easing Into Reading (decoding)
The Auditory Phonics Program (TAPP) (decoding)
Auditory Discrimination in Depth (decoding)

ATTENTION FOCUS
Synchronized Reading (with Neurological Impress)
Easing Into Reading (decoding)
The Auditory Phonics Program (TAPP) (decoding)
Auditory Discrimination in Depth (decoding)

As soon as symbol memory of three units is present, we begin working to develop a reading system. Once the individual can visually retain three symbols (numerals, letters, or shapes), then a letter symbol and its sound are introduced. With a three digit recall, the individual can support the recall and blending of two sounds. When they can recall four digits, then they have enough recall to be able to recognize three letter, phonetically consistent words.

Obviously, we need to pace the introduction of combinations of letters (words) to the individual's memory or digit recall system. This pacing assures success and allows the client to show long term retention. The digit recall should exceed the number of letters in the words by one digit for efficient processing. Once they have a six to eight unit (digit) automatic memory skill, they can usually retain words comfortably. This memory skill and the strategies for using it are necessary for both reading and spelling proficiency.

The beginning systems which we use for individuals who are non-readers or who read at third grade or below in testing are those listed under the Visual Symbol Confusion category above. Each of these systems teaches each symbol thoroughly and limits the presentation until the individual has learned it on an automatic basis. These systems also utilize a variety of strategies which are necessary in reading retention.

EASING INTO READING

Easing Into Reading program was a program which we developed over the past twenty-five years and has now been made available outside of our center. It was designed for individual or classroom use with students in first or second grade who were not learning through a traditional approach to reading.

The concepts which the program used were based on those which were important for teaching the individual with visual symbol confusion who had not been successful in learning a reading system. The program emphasized the following:

1. Each sound was presented with a multi-sensory approach.
2. Sounds were initially taught in isolation and no new sounds were presented until they were consistently competent with the previous sound.
3. Only one vowel sound was presented (short a) during the first sections of the program.
4. The sounds were matched with the symbol.
5. Only sound names were used, no alphabet labels.
6. Words were read very early in the program to provide immediate success.

The program activities in the beginning focused on introduction of the sounds for b, t, m and a. The tasks provided the student with good reinforcement of these sounds. Tasks included matching of sounds and symbols, rhythm patterns with sounds and symbols, tracking tasks, and practice in writing the symbols while verbalizing them.

These types of activities are easily developed by a creative instructor. The tasks include matching activities in which the symbol is shown at the left of a row and the student is asked to find matching symbols in the row. Each time the students see the symbol he verbalizes the sound for the symbol which reinforces the symbol to sound connection.

b	m	a	b	t	b
m	b	m	a	t	m

While they verbalize the sound, they should trace over the symbol with the index finger so that they are receiving tactile/kinesthetic feedback with each task. This reinforces the sound with the symbol and emphasizes the important rehearsal.

The same page may be used several times for the students. The task can be varied by having them do the page independently with a highlighter pen or even fold the stimulus column (left hand) back and have them study the sound/symbol and then turn the page over and match it. These types of tasks should initially be done with an instructor and then later can be an independent task.

A second type of task asks the students to work with the sounds in a rhythmic pattern. This reinforces a rhythm when verbalized and allows them to alternate between decoding and encoding activities. The page should have a pattern of sounds repeated several times.

b	a	b	_	b	a	_	a	b	_	b
m	b	m	b	_	b	m	_	m	_	m
a	b	m	_	b	m	a	_	m	a	_

On this page, they trace over the letters while making the sounds. When a line is completed the instructor may lead the students in a rhythmic chant of the sounds as they tap each symbol.

A third task has students working on tracking activities. In this activity, students verbalize the sound that they are tracking and trace the line from the sound to the same symbol on the other side of the maze. A separate color is used for each of the letters. Students enjoy this type of activity and it is helpful in improving fine motor coordination and developing visual tracking skills. The instructor may ask questions like. *"What color line did you choose for the "m" sound?"* or *"What sound did you connect with the red line?"*

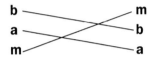

The first key for effectiveness in this reading program's approach is the consistent verbalization, tracing (tactile/kinesthetic stimulation) and discussion of the sounds as the students work. The second key is the repetition and reinforcement of work with the same sounds in a variety of activities. The third key is the instructor's comments of *"You read that very well."* As soon as students can say the sound with the symbol, they are complimented on their good reading skills.

The fourth task asks students to play with the sounds. The instructor may place the letter cards for the four sounds around the room. They are asked to locate the cards, but not to move them. They walk around the room locating the letter cards and remembering where they are located. They are then given a clue: *"on the desk"* or *"on the shelf"* or *"by the door"* and asked to give the sound which is nearest that location. This is a memory task which promotes spatial recall as well as visual symbol memory. Since it is a game, the students enjoy the task while they are developing important memory and reading skills.

The fifth task is a dictation activity. We usually call it a spelling test. We explain to the student that spelling is writing the symbol or symbols that you hear. During the first levels, the dictation may include single letter sounds and shapes. The dictation might include:

Teacher	Student Paper
1. "b"	1.
2. Make a diamond.	2.
3. "m"	3.
4. "t"	4.
5. Make a circle.	5.
6. "a" (short vowel sound)	6.

A later level of dictation may include two or three digit items for "spelling." It might look like this:

Teacher	Student Paper
1. "b" "a"	1.
2. circle "m"	2.
3. "t" "a"	3.
4. "m" "a" "t"	4.
5. "b" diamond	5.

As soon as these activities are comfortable for the students and they have a good recall of these symbols the focus moves to sound blending tasks with these same symbols. The matching task has a combination of the consonant sound and short vowel "a."

ba	ma	ba	ta	ab	ba
ta	ta	ba	am	at	ta

The pattern task also uses the blended syllable for the verbal rhythm coding. The students become comfortable in blending the syllables easily.

ma	ba	ma	_	ma	ba	_	ba	ma	ba
ta	ma	ba	ta	ma	_	ta	_	ba	ta

Dictation tasks use the same syllables for the students to spell. If any of the students are still experiencing challenges with closure on the sounds, the instructor may dictate the non-sense word with the sounds "b" "a" and then as a syllable "ba."

In addition to these tasks, the students should be asked to make their letters in three dimensional materials. A variety of materials have been used but play dough, clay, sand paper, felt or cardboard are most effective. Students are often asked to walk the letter pattern on the floor. The letter can be traced on the back of the students hand or student's back for additional tactile stimulation. This reinforces the pattern of the letter and creates the visual pattern. The training activities recommended under Spelling Development in this chapter which emphasize the development of visualization of the images should also be used.

The more stimulation students experience with the initial set of letters, the more effective they are in long term retention of reading symbols. The rehearsal of the sounds and symbols through many modes, in fact, stimulates the pathways in the brain and promotes learning and retention. This systematic approach to exercising each of the sensory areas required for reading assures long term success. Additional symbols are not added until students are very comfortable with these symbols/sounds and their formation. In some cases it may take several months for the first few symbols to be learned so that they are automatically accessible for the student. It is important that this "overlearning" take place before adding another symbol since this effort is creating the system of neurological paths for subsequent reading success.

We have found that this program can also be used with students who are inefficient or slow learners as well as those at risk for dyslexic frustration. Since these reading activities include extensive "overlearning" they promote retention of symbolic information. Once students have developed the learning pathways they become automatic learners. Their brains have been conditioned to learn symbolic information and make the verbal and motor match. They "know" how to learn symbolic information and are successful.

The sequence for introducing the sounds was carefully correlated with reading materials such as McGraw Hill Programmed Reading (Sullivan Series) which is referenced in the Appendix.

THE AUDITORY PHONICS PROGRAM (TAPP)

The Auditory Phonics Program was designed to model the Easing Into Reading effectiveness with strong sound/symbol training. It is effective with students from ages seven through adult. It is presented in a mature format so that adults who are non-readers can use the materials.

The program emphasizes the development of auditory discrimination, visual memory, sound sequencing, sound blending and sound/symbol integration skills. These are the essential reading elements which have been identified in research. The use of all the senses is emphasized to promote integrated learning. The program activities are similar to Easing Into Reading and provide considerable reinforcement to encourage individuals in retention of symbols. The components focus on the following:

1. The sounds are presented in a multi-sensory manner.
2. Sounds are presented in isolation and then in syllables to assist blending and closure skills.
3. Two short vowel sounds are introduced at the beginning of the program to assist in sound discrimination.
4. Syllables and words are read early in the program to reinforce reading success.

Individuals respond very effectively to the introduction of the sounds and we make no attempt in the beginning to introduce the letter name. In our experience, they appear to acquire the letter names when they are ready to make the association and we rarely find a need to teach the names. Important focus is kept on rehearsing the sounds and reinforcing them during the lesson. The activities parallel those described in the Easing Into Reading Program. The reference for program acquisition is included in the Appendix.

AUDITORY DISCRIMINATION IN DEPTH

Charles H. and Patricia C. Lindamood are the authors of the A.D.D. Program: Auditory Discrimination in Depth. These pioneers have provided a significant system for developing reading skills. The program meets the criteria which we find essential to success in developing reading skills. For our purposes, a successful reading system establishes the following:

1. Sound symbol association through a multi-sensory approach.
2. Thorough instruction of each sound with consistent repetition until it becomes part of an automatic system.
3. Integration from the auditory to visual channels. (Associating the sound to the symbol.)
4. Recognition that there are multiple sounds for some symbols.
5. Conceptualization of the sound including: feeling, hearing, seeing how it is made (mirror), seeing the symbol and associating it.

The A.D.D. Program begins with helping individuals understand the process which occurs in their brain as they are reading. Individuals learn what the brain looks like and what the major parts of the brain do to support learning. Then they learn about the pathways between learning areas and how the paths send messages from one area to another. Some of these can become permanent paths.

The A.D.D. Program was published originally in 1969 and

updated in 1975. It has been used for many years by speech and language therapists because of the effective manner in which it assisted in teaching sound production and discrimination. The student learns twenty-four consonant sounds and fifteen vowel sounds plus the r-controlled vowels.

Each sound is introduced with a label that describes how it is made. For instance a "p" sound is a "lip popper." This describes what it looks like when the individual makes the sound and looks in the mirror at the production. A picture card is provided for each of the consonant pairs or groups. The card has the letter symbol and a simple line drawing which depicts the mouth making the sound.

The A.D.D. Program can be learned by following the instructional manual available with the program from the reference in the Appendix. It is suggested that, if at all possible, teachers attend a training program to learn how to use the program most effectively. The skill of the presentation is essential in delivering the program in an interesting manner with the appropriate speed to maintain maximum progress and interest. This program is effective with all ages of students and we have found it equally effective for individual and group instruction.

ORTON GILLINGHAM TECHNIQUE

This technique is based on an integration of the senses used for reading and spelling. It is an excellent technique for developing all of the senses and bringing them together for reading and spelling. Anna Gillingham worked with Samuel Orton for two years in the Language Project of the New York Neurological Institute. She knew from her teaching experience that the systems which were commonly being used in classrooms were ineffective for some of the children who appeared bright and had good verbal skills. She developed a system for training teachers to use these techniques and become effective in producing readers.

The technique emphasizes the use of the senses in recognizing how a symbol (or word) looks, sounds, and feels (both in the speech organs as it is said and the hand as it is written). There are two associations that are essential in the teaching. The first is the development of the verbalization of the symbol or word through a Visual/Auditory/Kinesthetic (Speech) sequence. In this process the teacher displays the visual symbol, says the sound and the student repeats it. The student is encouraged to feel the speech organs as they repeat the sound so that they gain the kinesthetic experience, also.

The second type of linkage uses the Visual/Kinesthetic or written mode for reinforcement. In this task the student observes the teacher make a letter and then traces over the teacher's model. This is followed by a copying, writing from memory and finally writing from memory without looking at the stimulus. Once the student has learned through these systems then the linkages are reinforced with various drills.

This technique utilizes the multi-sensory approach which is so important for learning for the individual with a dyslexic learning style. There is a logical and detailed approach to presenting each of the letter sounds and many reinforcement activities which require the student to integrate learning through each of the senses. The reference by June L. Orton in the Materials and Program Appendix provides an excellent description of the method. Educators can receive additional training in the technique with classes based upon Slingerland's adaptation of these techniques. The references are provided in the appendix.

GLASS PERCEPTUAL DECODING SYSTEM

Individuals who would benefit from a visual approach to learning to read are often successful with Gerald G. Glass' program for "perceptual conditioning for decoding." Dr. Glass feels that the decoding process is an essential part of learning to read. He uses the analogy *"Hearing is to listening as decoding is to reading"* to emphasize the importance of this skill.

This system breaks down the reading process into visual and auditory clustering. Glass has found that good readers are conditioned to recognize the "clusters" in words. This skill enables them to recognize new words which have similar clusters to known words. This system insists that the individual recognize the clusters within words. Therefore, they are consistently presented with whole words and work on exploring the clusters within the word.

When individuals either have learned or already know the sounds in words, we find that they can benefit from using the Glass techniques. It has been especially helpful when they are having challenges in transitioning from sounding out and blending sounds to recognizing whole words. These techniques promote the skills for whole word recognition.

Our observations in working with numerous individuals using this technique is that it not only teaches reading as a system but it improves visual memory skills. They need to be able to use their visual retention skills at a five unit memory level in order to be successful. At that level we find that their memory actually increases with the practice of the perceptual clusters.

Glass has published work books which reinforce the acquisition of the sound clusters. This program is included in the references in the Materials and Programs Appendix. This system is quite effective and should be a part of the variety of techniques that an instructor has for teaching reading systems.

ADDITIONAL READING SYSTEMS
The Neurological Impress Reading program and Synchronized Reading are both discussed in Chapter 9. These systems are important for assisting the individual who has some basic reading skills, but has challenges in comprehension and comfort in

reading. They are especially useful for improving learning for the individual with **Auditory Comprehension** or **Attention Focus Confusion** learning styles.

COMPREHENSION TRAINING

There are many materials which provide assistance in improving comprehension skills. The important part of training comprehension skills is in recognizing the elements associated with understanding and in teaching these. We recognize two levels of comprehension needs: Comprehension for casual or pleasure reading and comprehension for studying or acquisition of technical information.

The first level of comprehension is usually that which is needed for reading a novel, magazine article or even reading an instruction or recipe. For this level of comprehension the Neurological Impress Reading is very effective. The client finds that the information is retained with minimum effort.

The second level of comprehension training is that which enables the individual to read for gaining technical information, analysis of literature, report writing and other skills needed for success in junior high school through university work. This training requires the individual to have skills in recognizing the main idea, support statements, responding to a variety of types of questions from factual to inference.

For the second level of comprehension the materials which are provided in study skill programs, Barnell Loft, Reading for Concepts and others give organized graded programs. These programs are referenced in the Materials and Programs Appendix.

The important aspect of teaching advanced comprehension skills is to "actively" teach them. If we give the individual a selection to read and then have them answer the questions included with the program we are **not teaching** we are **testing**. There is a major difference in the progress and the motivation individuals have toward the activity. When we teach with the materials we constantly work with the strategies for how to do the task.

For instance, if the skill is learning to recognize the main idea in a paragraph we need to structure the task. We guide them in exploring by rephrasing the question until it is understood. For instance, instead of saying *"Find the main idea,"* we might say *"Do you have any idea what this story is about?"... "What clues can you find that might tell you what this paragraph is going to tell us?"* The clues that they will need to use will be the title, pictures, previous paragraph, etc. Teach them to explore all of these clues. Prompt them to experience the clues if they have not yet learned to recognize them.

Many individuals find that they benefit from using a who/what/when/where/how/why exploration technique to improve their comprehension. With this technique they are prompted to read a sentence or several sentences for the purpose of identifying "who" it is talking about. The specific focus on one element of the selection narrows it sufficiently to allow comprehension success and provide a guide for the reader.

As readers mature in comprehending they find that they are automatically identifying these components in a selection. The information begins to make sense because of the structure which they are bringing to it.

One additional activity which we find very effective involves having the reader image what they are reading. This is especially effective when it is broken down into the components of who/what/where. When a descriptive sentence is read they are asked what the character might have looked like. They are encouraged to "see" the person with their imagination. In the early stages of this activity they may need the assistance of reading materials which have illustrations. This will provide the image of the character in a concrete manner.

As they become skilled in using their imagery they will find they enjoy imaging the character without illustrations.

Learning to image information as it is heard or read is an excellent skill. It improves memory for long-term retention and can be used for acquiring complex concepts with minimal effort.

These *active* teaching techniques are most convenient on a one-to-one basis but can be readily adapted to a reading group. The instructor can teach strategies to the group in the same manner. The instructor will just need to monitor the different levels of success with each student and adapt their questioning technique appropriately.

The important aspect of "teaching" something is breaking it down into the parts which will lead to success. This analysis is critical in teaching the strategies which allow successful comprehension. Each of the techniques which have been presented here break things down into their simple elements and therefore, lead to success.

Individuals who experience auditory comprehension confusion need to learn the strategies which allow them to understand what they are reading. The combination of improved memory skills, language development, and both the decoding and comprehension systems will promote their success with reading.

SPELLING –NEUROLOGICAL IMPRESS

Many individuals with the Visual Symbol Confusion learning style experience serious challenges in developing spelling skills. They frequently have difficulty in recalling the visual image of the word and usually do not realize how to hold visual symbol information effectively. Their spelling skills often have difficulty going above the third grade level.

The Neurological Impress Spelling method is effective in teaching spelling for individuals with the dyslexic learning style. It utilizes a multi-sensory approach and provides for active use of memory skills. The following steps are utilized in learning a word:

1. Say the word and discuss the meaning of it prior to looking at the word. It is important that the individual have a visual image of the meaning of the word. If the word is "bread," talk about the different meanings of the word. Most individuals will be familiar with the word bread as used in making a sandwich. Explore other meanings such as: bread which means one's livelihood, *"I am the bread winner in the family."*; or to put crumbs on something, *"I will bread the pork chops."*

   Ask individuals to form a visual image using the concept and tell you about it. If they have not already done so, have them give you a sentence using the word.

2. Write the word on a card, use cursive or manuscript writing, whichever is more familiar for them.

3. Ask them to trace over the letters with a colored marker, crayon or pen and say the letters as they are traced.

4. Have them look at the word until they feel they can image it on the wall when they look up. Let them tell you when they are ready.

5. Ask them to image the word on the wall and then show you where they have placed it by tracing over the image and saying the letters at the same time.

At this point there are several different ways to "rehearse" the word. We will share these for use either separately or in combinations:

Activity I

1. Explore the word from the projected image with them and have them point to the last letter of the word and

say it. Point to the first letter of the word. Point to the letter next to the b. Point to the middle letter.
2. Ask them to spell the word from the image on the wall.
3. Ask them to image the word on a paper and trace over it.

Activity II

1. Explore the word rom the projected image with the student. Have them point to each letter and say it.
2. Ask the student to trace over the first two letters and tell you what they are. Then have them take the next three letters and move them to the wall on their right. Ask the student to trace over them and tell you what they are.
3. Ask the student to take the first two letters and move them to the floor in front of them. Have the student say what the letters are. Next have the student take the other letters and put them in place with the first letters on the floor. Have them spell the whole word and point to the letters as they do.
4. Have the student pick up the word and put it on the paper in front of themselves. Ask the student to trace over the word and spell it for you.

These exercises of visual memory are quite effective. Students are working with the word from memory through each of the tasks. Reinforcement is provided through the visualization, verbalization and tactile/kinesthetic rehearsal. It is not unusual for an individual to be willing to work with a word for several minutes by moving it around the room and putting it in different places. If they are young and need to be active, individuals can get up and write it with a finger on the wall and physically "pretend" to carry it to different places like under the chair, on the shelf, in a book, or on the wall.

This technique is easily used for home practice of the spelling words. The words remain in memory far longer than with rehearsal purely by repetitious writing of the word or completing the fill in the blanks in a traditional speller. Meaning and understanding what the word is, visualization, verbal reinforcement and writing are all emphasized. Once the word has been introduced, then they can engage in a review or practice using memory skills as follows:

Activity III

1. Ask the individuals to fold a piece of lined paper in half lengthwise. Have them number the columns 1 and 2 on the two columns on the front side and 3 and 4 on the back side.
2. Have them look at the spelling word on the card. When they feel that they have the image of the word, have them turn the card over and write the word in the first column from their visual image.
3. Ask them to check the spelling to be certain it is correct.
4. Ask them to fold the paper in half and look at the word in the first column until they can retain the image. Then turn over the paper and write it in the second column . Open the paper and check the spelling. Continue this activity through third and fourth columns.

The benefit of practicing the word in this manner is that each time they correctly image the word and they have to use memory skills to write it. This engages an active memory process which is most likely to remain for long term recall.

The other benefit of this technique is that it trains individuals to begin imaging words as they are seeing them. When they are reading and seeing words over and over the words will begin to be "impressed" for later use in writing and spelling. This is the mode with which we really learn to develop spelling vocabulary. The exposure to words with repetition develops and extends our spelling vocabulary.

The frequently used method of writing words ten times (or more) is far less effective because it does not recall active use of memory. In fact, many students practice their words letter by letter when asked to write words ten times. They write b, b, b, b, b, b, b followed by placing the r, r, r, r, r, etc. next to the b for br on their way to having ten copies of the word "bread"! Classroom teachers who use the four column spelling practice method for teaching spelling find that their children remember the words longer and are less resistant to practicing.

One caution in teaching spelling. Individuals will only learn words and retain them if they have adequate visual memory skills. When a client can recall five or more units of visual information, then they can work on four and five letter words. They should be retaining six to seven units before they can handle multi-syllable words. At that point, they will engage in clustering or chunking the information and can be successful.

EXPECTATIONS FOR LEARNING

These reading and spelling systems are effective for individuals with the dyslexic learning style. A skilled instructor will learn to use the different systems and recognize when to use some of the strategies from one system to augment another. Most individuals with unique learning styles will learn to read within a period of eight to twenty months. Even clients who come in as mature adults starting at a symbol recognition level, will find that they can develop a system for reading and spelling. The combination of developing processing skills, establishing strategies for effective use of talents and skills and a comfortable system for reading equals success for the individual with a dyslexic learning style.

Materials and Programs Appendix

Basta, J. & Smith, J.M. (1973) *Ready, Set, Go For Language Competency.* Sacramento, CA: Learning Time Publications. (7230 S. Land Park Drive, #101, Sacramento, CA 95831).

Bauman, B. (1979) *Super Reader.* (How to Teach Your Child to Speed Read) Briarcliff Manor, NY: Stein and Day. (Briarcliff Manor, NY 10510).

Belgau, F.A. (1971) *Activities for the Development of Perceptual Motor and Visual Perception Skills.* (Training Program) Port Angeles, WA: Balametrics, Inc.

Boder, E. & Jarrico, S. (1982) *The Boder Test of Reading Spelling Patterns.* (Diagnostic Screening Test for Subtypes of Reading Disabilities) New York: Grune & Stratton, Inc., (111 Fifth Avenue, New York, NY 10003).

Davis, R. *Davis Orientation Mastery Training.* (In-service Training services) Burlingame, CA: Reading Research Council. (1799 Old Bayshore Highway, Suite 248, Burlingame, CA 94010).

Dennison, P. & Dennison, G. (1989) *Brain Gym: Teacher's Edition.* (Manual to Explain, Instruct and Facilitate Movement Activities for Whole Brain Learning) Glendale, CA: Edu/Kinesthetics, Inc. (P O Box 5002, Glendale, CA 91201).

Dunn, L.M. & Smith, J.O. (1966) *Peabody Language Development Kit.* (Kit and manual) Circle Pines, MN: American Guidance Service, Inc. (Publisher's Building, Circle Pines, MN 55014).

Frostig, M. & Maslow, P. (1973) *Learning Problems in the Classroom.* (Text on Prevention and Remediation of Learning Problems) San Francisco, CA: Grune & Stratton, A Subsidiary of Harcourt, Brace, Jovanovich.

Glass, G.G. *Perceptual Conditioning for Decoding.* (Reading method and materials) Garden City, NY: Easier to Learn Materials. (PO Box 329, Garden City, NY 11530).

Greene, L. & Jones-Baman, L. (1985) *Getting Smarter.* (Study skills reference) Belmont, CA: David S. Lake.

Haag, C., Ironside, R.A., Nagel, R.E., Cross, A.R., Sayles, D.G. & Valusek, J.E. (1961) *Learning to Learn.* (Study skills reference) New York: Harcourt, Brace, Jovanovich.

Hammill, D.D. (1985) *Detroit Test of Learning Aptitude.* (Assessment Instrument) Novato, CA: Academic Therapy Publications.

Heckelman, R. G. (1966) *Using the Neurological Impress Reading Technique. Academic Therapy*, Vol. 1, Summer, 1966.

Jastak, S. & Wilkinson, G.S. (1984) *Wide Range Achievement Test R.* (Academic Assessment Instrument) Wilmington, Delware: Jastak Assessment Systems Jastak Associates, Inc. (1526 Gilpin Avenue, Wilmington, Delware, 19806).

Kaufman, A.S. & Kaufman, N.L. (1983) *Kaufman Assessment Battery for Children.* (Academic Assessment Instrument) Circle Pines, MN: American Guidance Services. (Publisher's Building, Circle Pines, MN 550141796).

Lindamood, C.H. & Lindamood, P.C. (1979) *Auditory Discrimination in Depth.* (Reading program kit) Austin, TX: (Pro-Ed,, 8700 Shoal Creek Boulevard, Austin, TX 78757-6897).

Markwardt, F.C. (1989) *Peabody Individual Achievement Test R.* (Academic Assessment Instrument) Circle Pines, Minn: American Guidance Service, Inc. (Publisher's Building, Circle Pines, MN 55014-1796).

Marolda, M (1976) *Attribute Games and Problems.* (Attribute Materials and Blocks) Nashua, NH: (Delta Education, Inc. P. O. Box 3000, Nashua, HH 03061-991).

Critical Thinking Press & Software (Logic, reasoning, verbal and figural thinking skills materials) Pacific Grove, CA: (PO Box 448, Pacific Grove, CA 93950-4849).

Roach, E.G. & Kephart, N.C. (1966) *Purdue Perceptual Motor Survey.* (Perceptual/motor Assessment Instrument) San Antonio, TX: Charles Merrill Books, Inc. & The Psychological Corporation.

Slingerland, B.H. *Screening Test for Identifying Children with Specific Language Disability.* (Assessment Instrument) Cambridge, MA: Educators Publishing Service. (75 Moulton Street, Cambridge, MA 022389101).

Smith, J.M. (1991) *Easing Into Reading Program.* (Reading materials for beginning phonic development for young students) Sacramento, CA: Learning Time Publications. (7230 S. Land Park Drive, #101, Sacramento, CA 95831).

Smith, J.M. (1978) *Melvin-Smith Receptive Expressive Observation.* (Memory and Processing Assessment Instrument) Sacramento, CA: Learning Time Publications. (7230 S. Land Park Drive, #101,, Sacramento, CA, 95831).

Smith, J. M. (1993) *The Auditory Phonics Program.* (Reading materials for beginning phonic development for older students.) Sacramento, CA: Learning Time Publications. (7230 S. Land Park Drive, #101, Sacramento, CA 95831).

St. John, J. *Project PRES.* (Newsletter for Acupressure in the Classroom) Santa Cruz, CA: Santa Cruz County Office of Education. (809H Bay Avenue, Capitola, CA 95010).

Sutphin, F. (1967) *A Perceptual Testing and Training Handbook for First Grade Teachers.* (Perceptual training program) Winter Haven, FL: Winter Haven Lions Research Foundation, Inc.

Woodcock, R.W. & Johnson, M.B. (1977) *Woodcock Johnson Psycho/Educational Battery.* (Academic Assessment Instrument) Hingham, MA: Teaching Resources. (50 Pond Park Road, Hingham, MA 02043).

ASSESSMENT BATTERY

Smith, J.M. (1996) Competency Assessment Battery–CAB (Computerized assessment battery for processing, attention and academic skill measurement) Sacramento, CA: Learning Time Publications. (7230 S. Land Park Drive, #101, Sacramento, CA 95831).

Endnotes

CHAPTER 1

1. Melvin-Smith Learning Center, 7230 South Land Park Drive, Suite 101, Sacramento, CA 95831. (916) 392-6415

CHAPTER 2

1. Reading Research Council, 1799 Old Bayshore Highway, Suite 248, Burlingame, CA 94010. (415) 6928990.

CHAPTER 5

1 Richard T. Thieriot, Editorials: "Appalling Illiteracy," *San Francisco Chronicle.* (1988, May 22).

2. Ellen Hawkes, "I Had to Grow Up Fast," *Parade Magazine* (1989, January 8): 1213.

3. Bob Dart, "Manley's Secret Shame," *Cox Newspapers,* Reprinted in the *San Francisco Chronicle* (1988, May).

4. Karen Berney, "Can Your Workers Read?" *Nation's Business* (1988, October): 2530.

5. Federal Register, P.L. 94142, The Education for All Handicapped Children Act of 1975.

Bibliography

Ayres, A. Jean. *Sensory Integration and Learning Disorders.* Los Angeles: Western Psychological Services, 1972.

Berney, Karen. "Can Your Workers Read?" *Nation's Business.* October 1988: 2530.

Boder, E. *The Boder Test of Reading/Spelling Patterns: A Diagnostic Screening Test for Subtypes of Reading Disability.* New York: Gruene & Stratton, 1982.

Critchley. *The Dyslexic Child.* London: Wm. Heinemann Medical Book Ltd.., 1970.

Dart, Bob. "Manley's Secret Shame." *Cox Newspapers.* Reprinted in the San Francisco Chronicle. May 1988.

Davis, R. The Gift of Dyslexia. Burlingame, CA: Ability Workshop Press. (Reading Research Council).

Duffy, F.H., et al. "Dyslexia: Regional Differences in Brain Electrical Activity by Topographical Mapping." *Annals of Neurology*, 7. 5 (1979): 412420.

Galaburda, A.M. *Development Dyslexia: A Review of Biological Interactions.* Reprint 105. Baltimore, MD: The Orton Dyslexia Society, 1989.

Hawkes, Ellen. "I Had to Grow Up Fast." *Parade Magazine.* 8 January 1989: 1213.

Hynd, G.W. and C. Hynd. "Dyslexia: Neuroanatomical/Neurolinguistic Perspectives." *Reading Research Quarterly, XIX.* (1984): 482498.

Hynd, G.W., et al. "Regional Cerebral Blood Flow (RCBF) in Developmental Dyslexia: Activation During Reading in a Surface and Deep Dyslexic." *Journal of Learning Disabilities, 20.* 5 (1987): 295299.

Johnson, D. and H. Myklebust. *Learning Disabilities: Educational Principles and Practices.* New York: Gruene & Stratton, 1967.

Levinson, H. *Smart But Feeling Dumb.* New York: Warner Books, Inc., 1984.

Naour P.J. and D.J. Martin. *Developmental Component in Brain Electrical Activity of Normal and Learning Disabled Boys.* Paper presented at the Annual Meeting of the American Educational Research Association. Montreal, Canada, April 1983.

Orton, June L. "The Orton Gillingham Approach." Reprinted from *The Disabled Reader: Education of the Dyslexic Child.* Baltimore, Maryland: John Hopkins Press, 1966.

Rawson, M. B. "The Nature of the Dyslexic Learner." *Proceedings of the Orton Dyslexia Society Symposium: Dyslexia and Evolving Educational Patterns.* 1014.

Shaywitz, B. and S. Waxman. "Dyslexia." *The New England Journal of Medicine,* 316. 20 1987: 12681270.

Thieriot, Richard T. "Appalling Illiteracy." Editorial. *San Francisco Chronicle.* 22 May 1988.

Torello M.W. and F. H. Duffy. "Using Brain Electrical Mapping to Diagnose Learning Disabilities." *Theory Into Practice*, 24. 2 (1985): 9599.

United States. Federal Register." The Education for All Handicapped Children Act of 1975." P.L. 94142.

Program and Content Guide

REFERENCE:
CHAPTER 8 - PREPARING THE BRAIN
FOR LEARNING

CHAPTER 9 - STRATEGIES THAT WORK

CHAPTER 10 - READING STRATEGIES THAT WORK